THE SIMPLE LIFE

GUIDE TO OPTIMAL HEALTH

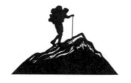

Other Books by Gary Collins

Going Off The Grid: The How-To Book of
Simple Living and Happiness

Living Off The Grid: What to Expect While Living
the Life of Ultimate Freedom and Tranquility

The Beginners Guide To Living Off The Grid:
The DIY Workbook for Living the Life You Want

The Simple Life Guide to RV Living: The Road to Freedom
and the Mobile Lifestyle Revolution

The Simple Life Guide To Decluttering Your Life:
The How-To Book of Doing More with Less
and Focusing on the Things That Matter

For a complete and updated list of *The Simple Life* book series and
other books by Gary Collins, go to **www.thesimplelifenow.com**.

THE *SIMPLE LIFE*

GUIDE TO OPTIMAL HEALTH

How to Get Healthy and Feel
Better Than Ever

GARY COLLINS, MS

The Simple Life Series (Book 2)

The Simple Life Guide to Optimal Health: How to Get Healthy and Feel Better Than Ever

First Edition

Printed in the United States of America

Copyright ©2018

Published by Second Nature Publishing, Albuquerque, NM 87109

For information about special discounts for bulk purchasing, and/or direct inquiries about copyright, permission, reproduction and publishing inquiries, please contact Book Publishing Company at 888-260-8458.

DISCLAIMER OF WARRANTY

The information contained in this material may not be appropriate for everyone, particularly for anyone suffering from any disease or recovering from a physical injury. Any time you intend to make a change in your nutrition or exercise program consult with your physician for guidance and to gain clearance to participate in such a program. The intent of this information is to further educate you in the area of nutrition and physical exercise, not to diagnose, treat, or cure any physical, mental, or any other conditions that should be under the advisement of a doctor.

Statements contained in this product have not been evaluated by the Food and Drug Administration (FDA). None of the products or services offered in this material are intended to diagnose, treat, cure or prevent any disease.

The text included in this material is for informational purposes only. The data and information contained herein are based upon information from various published and unpublished sources that represent training, health and nutrition literature and practice summarized by the authors and publisher. Even though the authors have been as thorough as possible in their research, the publisher of this text makes no warranties, expressed or implied, regarding the currency, completeness, or scientific accuracy of this information, nor does it warrant the fitness of the information for any particular purpose. Any claims or presentations regarding any specific products or brand names are strictly the responsibility of the product owners or manufacturers. This summary of information from unpublished sources, books, research journals, and articles is not intended to replace the advice or attention of health care professionals. It is not intended to direct their behavior or replace their independent professional judgment.

ISBN 978-1-57067-383-2

Get Your Free Goodies and Stuff!

Building a solid relationship with my readers is very important to me. It is one of the rewards of being a writer. From time to time, I send out my newsletter (never spammy, I promise) to keep you up to date with special offers and information about anything new I may be doing.

If that's not enough enticement, when you sign up for my newsletter I'll send you some spectacular free stuff!

1. Gary's three-day fat blast

2. Gary's current workout routine

3. Beginner grocery shopping list

You can get all the goodies above by signing up for my mailing list at: **www.thesimplelifenow.com/healthyresources**.

TABLE OF CONTENTS

INTRODUCTION: What Is This Book About?   9

1 My Journey to Health   13

2 Getting Back to Basics   20

3 The Five Principles of
The Simple Life Healthy Lifestyle Plan   23

4 Addressing Today's Common Health Myths   30

5 Why It Takes Guts to Be Healthy   36

6 Why Are We Addicted to Refined Carbohydrates?   44

7 Does Eating Fat Make You Fat?   66

8 Tackling the Cholesterol Myth   90

9 The Importance of Protein in
Maintaining a Healthy Weight   104

10 Is Counting Calories Important?   136

11 Your Body Is an Ocean—Understanding
Proper Water and Salt Consumption   144

12 Sleep Yourself to Health   155

13 Stress—the Silent Killer 160

14 You've Gotta Move! Exercise 101 164

15 Should I Take Supplements
in Order to Be Healthy? 188

16 Intermittent Fasting and the Ketogenic State 198

17 *The Simple Life Healthy Lifestyle*
Starter Grocery Shopping List 205

18 *The Simple Life Healthy Lifestyle*
Starter Recipes 211

ABOUT GARY 245

REFERENCES 247

INTRODUCTION

What Is This Book About?

In this book I want to introduce you to what I like to call *The Simple Life Healthy Lifestyle Plan*. This all-encompassing lifestyle plan is something I put together after decades of being a special agent for the U.S. Department of Health and Human Services and U.S. Food and Drug Administration, and after working with thousands of clients in the realm of health and wellness.

What I have learned from working with clients, and from working on my own health, is that most people today feel terrible but they have no idea where to start when it comes to bettering their health and wellness. There are thousands of health books, all touting instant health, and endless internet websites and blogs making it more confusing than ever before. Here's a simple fact: People today are buying more health-related cookbooks than at any point in our history, but the irony is fewer people are cooking their own meals and many are the unhealthiest they've ever been. Hmm, something is wrong here!

I can tell you from the insider perspective of someone who has worked deep inside the food, drug and health industries, it is not by accident. Here's the key, though: We can continue to blame everyone else, but the fact of the matter is there's one thing we have a lot of control of in our life: our health. No one is twisting your arm making you eat that doughnut and consume that thousand-calorie latte while sitting on the couch. The only person doing that is you.

I understand most people are lost when it comes to health, so that's where this book in my *The Simple Life* series comes in: to give you the right information to help fix the problem. Once you have the right information, you'll be surprised how easy being healthy really is . . . heck, how much easier life is in general. Say goodbye to those fad diets, magazine articles and TV shows touting the next miracle product or exercise and nutrition plan. Wouldn't you rather spend your time doing something else and saving your money? Most of those snake oil products make you lose weight in one place only: your wallet.

If you're reading this, it's probably because you want to change your life and be healthier.

Maybe you're already fit but want to take your health program to the next level.

Or maybe you're like most other Americans: You're really out of shape and want to be energetic and lean and look good in a bathing suit, but you just can't seem to get motivated.

The truth is, to change your life even a little, you'll need to take action. It does absolutely no good to learn about your health and do nothing.

The harder truth is you're going to have to get uncomfortable in the short term to be fit and to reach your ultimate health goals in the long run. The good news is, once you get there, it will be much easier to maintain a healthy body and spirit than you imagine now. Plus, you're not alone. Consider me your new health coach, here to help you from the comfort and privacy of your own home.

No matter where you start, this book has been written for you: to inspire, motivate and inform.

To this day, I have never had one person who has implemented my philosophy **NOT** succeed and become healthier. I consider optimal health and wellness to be the cornerstone of obtaining *The Simple Life*. Trust me, your life is a heck of a lot simpler when you're healthy. I know from personal experience, as I've changed my own health for the better and am now more productive and much, much happier than I was before. Isn't that what living *The Simple Life* is all about?

I want you to do great things and reach your fullest potential. Now let's get started.

1

My Journey to Health

This is my story. Although, legally, I can't tell all of it.

As a former special agent for the U.S. Department of Health and Human Services, and U.S. Food and Drug Administration, I am restricted from revealing specific details of investigations not already in the public record. But let's just say that what you don't know about how the health, food and drug industries work could definitely hurt you.

Through the years, I've felt a growing desire to share the information and knowledge I have to help people achieve their health goals and to live a healthy and fit life. I'm not some marketing guru or someone who decided that I wanted to get into the health business to dupe people and make money; I've spent decades as an avid athlete, personal trainer, health consultant, and an investigator in the realm of health and wellness. Bottom line: no one else in the health industry has my background—no one!

Here's how it all started for me.

If you're anything like me, you didn't spend the majority of your life knowing the best way to be healthy. For me, it took many years to assemble all the requisite pieces of the puzzle: diet, exercise, and insider knowledge about the health care and food industries.

Like many of you, my childhood sporting endeavors were largely fueled by sugary cereals, sweetened drinks, processed cheese-and-mayonnaise sandwiches, and other nutrient-free non-real-food concoctions. This was also the way all my friends ate, rich or poor. Yet almost all of us were skinny. I mean *really* skinny. How was this possible with such lackluster nutrition? Simply put, we ran around and played almost nonstop. Thus, we all burned huge amounts of calories.

Yet we also frequently came down with strange ailments. Often we didn't feel well, since we were calorie-rich but nutrient-deprived. If we hadn't exercised as much as we did, I'm sure we would have been overweight and less healthy. I look back now and realize I had no idea of how to eat well, or of the importance of avoiding extreme, quick-fix type diets and workout plans. I had been taught the usual carbohydrate-heavy, low-fat approach to eating and thought that, plus sports, was all I needed to be fit for life.

My misguided approach continued in college, where I tried various over-the-top ways to gain muscle mass. Instead of eating well, I focused only on how many calories I was taking in. I exercised at what I now see were inappropriate levels of intensity. My unhealthy approach left me exhausted and ill, especially when playing the sports I loved.

I majored in criminology, but also took various classes in health studies along the way. After working in the warehouse of a multinational food company (a brief stint that stirred the beginnings of my interest in the origins of our everyday food), I joined the U.S. military.

Back then in the military, we ate cafeteria-style food every day. If you've never done that, I'm here to tell you, don't start. That, coupled with the harsh and rigorous physical training for my military role, led to multiple long-term injuries.

That damage would later teach me to be cautious with my personal training clients—I know now that the exercise you perform should work *with* your body, not against it. This is a lesson I wish someone had taught me back then. My whole focus was on fitness; I was too inexperienced to recognize the value of *wellness* just yet.

Even as I served our country, my dual interests of forensic investigations and wellness were a part of my daily life. I worked as a cryptologist and also worked as a physical trainer for various military personnel. But I wanted to take my investigative interests to the next level. So when the opportunity arose, I completed a master's degree in forensic science. This led to my first non-military law enforcement job as a special agent for the U.S. State Department Diplomatic Security Service.

I subsequently became a special investigative agent for the FDA (Food and Drug Administration) and the HHS (Department of Health and Human Services). My work included investigating health care fraud, tainted food, prescription drug counterfeiting, the illegal importation of medical drugs, and other systemic and patient abuses.

My work as a special agent was stressful and demanding, frequently taking me around the world to far-flung locations of dubious repute. These voyages opened my eyes to how other cultures viewed food and health—often in much different (and more successful) ways than I had ever observed in America.

During my career I investigated a broad spectrum of health care providers, from purveyors of backroom "miracle" cures to the most respected of medical doctors (some of whom were doing very unrespectable things). To say that some of the activities that even "top" doctors are up to are shocking would be an understatement. Let's just say these insider experiences quickly convinced me of the importance of taking preventative wellness measures to avoid the need for later medical "care."

Fortunately, my investigations also involved many wellness-focused, non-M.D. professionals. So, oddly enough, it was my role with the FDA that introduced me to the concepts of natural eating and healing. Now there are certainly a lot of nefarious snake oil sellers out there, don't get me wrong. But there were also many reputable wellness-based professionals with alternative healing approaches that helped me rethink what I thought I knew about being fit.

It was then that I realized my skills as an investigator could be used to finally find the missing link between popular fitness programs and natural healing to really understand how to lose weight and be healthy in the long term, and within the broken systems of today's food supplies and healthcare.

Thus the seeds of *The Simple Life Healthy Lifestyle Plan* were sown. In my spare time I began my study of wellness and holistic healing in earnest.

It was, for a while, a dual life. By day I investigated dietary supplement fraud for the FDA; by night I studied the benefits of genuine, high-quality supplements. At work I saw how a misguided public is duped by the food industry, corporate marketing and even the government. So I used my professional skills as an investigator to scour medical journals and scientific research to find the missing piece in the nation's wellness equation.

Finally, the time was right to bring my experience and inside knowledge to light.

The questionable practices I witnessed in my previous FDA work inspired me to start my own company to share what I had learned. Now instead of quietly documenting all that goes wrong with our nation's food and supplement supplies, I am proactive and talk about health and the positive aspects of quality supplements.

Instead of relying on the muzzled investigators of a federal agency, I want everyday people to make informed decisions based on information that has, until now, been routinely hidden from public view.

My new mission in life is to bring such information to light. This is at the core of *The Simple Life Healthy Lifestyle Plan*.

Chances are, if you bought this book you are ready for a change. There's no shortage of health and diet fads out there—some more sane than others. Presumably, if they all offered the keys to the slim-and-slender kingdom, we would all be lean and healthy, right? Yet more Americans are overweight and unhealthy than ever before. Most Americans cannot even cook for themselves, thus the popularity of pre-prepared meals and meal ingredients with cooking instructions shipped in boxes to your door. This is not convenience or simplicity, this is pure laziness and being misguided on what actions to take to be healthy. Something is clearly missing.

Recently there's been a surge of investigative-style journalism focusing on the corporatization of America's formerly nutritious food supply. An industrial food machine has taken the place of America's bread basket, as animals and plants alike are mistreated, artificially stimulated, and even genetically modified so massive corporate entities can make more money, regardless of the appalling health consequences for you and your children.

Finally, the terrible truth about the man-made degradation of our soils, foods and farming traditions is filtering into the light. Interest in natural foods is likewise coming to the fore; organic foods are increasingly popular, and interest in preventative wellness measures is on the rise.

Yet there is a dearth of information that combines these concepts. On one end of the spectrum are books that describe the failings of our food supply. On the other end are the books that focus on natural and holistic ways of eating. The former are often entirely journalistic and theoretical, the latter, intimidating and frequently lacking in any exercise advice.

Until now.

I created *The Simple Life Healthy Lifestyle Plan* to address what I see as a lack of accurate, harmonious, integrity-based information for people who want to lose weight the right way—for good, and for life.

Overcoming My Own Resistance

Find it hard to get motivated?

I want you to understand you are not alone. I have also struggled over the years with my health.

About 12 years ago I was drinking too much alcohol and eating a lot of processed foods, and my health suffered because of this. At the time I was living in a very cold climate and kept telling myself that after winter I would get back into it—it was just too cold to go run or exercise right then. I was taking the easy way out and I knew it.

Finally, I convinced myself to stop making excuses and to get out there and take action. I remember there was a little snow on the ground and the wind was blowing. It was probably 30 degrees outside. In this dark and gloomy weather, my inner thoughts reminded me of how nice and warm my house was. All I had to do was go back inside.

But I took that first stride. I froze my butt off for the first mile, but once my body warmed up I started to feel better and better. Once I broke through that mental barrier, it was no longer such a struggle. I didn't notice how cold it was anymore. Every time I would make it back to my house after a run in the cold, with my nose red and runny and my ears freezing, I would look in the mirror and smile. What a sense of accomplishment.

I still look back at those winter runs with fond memories of the tranquility and therapeutic effects they brought me. Now, you don't necessarily need to go run in freezing weather to start your journey to optimal health, but you must mentally prepare yourself for the first step. It will be the hardest one you will take.

There are going to be days when you'd rather pick up some chicken nuggets and sit on the couch and watch TV instead of preparing a healthy meal and heading to the gym. Everyone has done this at some point, including myself.

From here on in, you will have to climb mountains you never thought you could climb. You are going to stumble at times. Just keep climbing.

And above all, don't give up!

2

Getting Back to Basics

The secrets of health and longevity today are the same as they were thousands of years ago for our prehistoric ancestors. This idea is at the heart of *The Simple Life* concept.

While we have many creature (and culinary!) comforts in our modern lives, our bodies and digestive systems have changed little since our prehistoric cousins found the secret to life-long health: active lives and natural foods. So we need to eat and move like they did. It doesn't get simpler than that!

This is not to say you need to live like a caveman—far from it! Hey, I don't want to give up my car or computer either...OK, maybe some days. But when it comes to your body, realize that the ideal diet and movement patterns that kept our species alive and empowered for many millennia haven't changed much.

Anytime you're confronted by a seemingly confusing health choice, just think of how your primitive brethren would have lived: with whole natural foods and an active lifestyle. Humans evolved consuming a diet of natural foods based on actively gathering plant-based foods and hunting animals. Our bodies, though highly adaptive, need specific nutrients that can only be found in nature to function properly. This has been the case for millions of years, and for far longer than our modern ways of eating have existed. This nutritional paradigm has only changed in the last few hundred years, thanks to the advent of industrialized agriculture and factory food production.

The prehistoric man/woman concept is an easy tool to use when you become confused about food, exercise or health choices. If the modern world as we know it were to end and you had to live off of the land like our predecessors, what would you eat? What foods would you have access to in your immediate area?

Whenever you have a question about your food selections, just imagine what a prehistoric man or woman would have had as food choices. Would they have had access to sugary flavored water, processed starchy pasta, high fructose corn syrup, sugary breakfast cereals, or artificial sweeteners? Did prehistoric man/woman worry about saturated fat? Humans before us did not concern themselves with counting calories or with most of our other modern dietary concerns. They just ate what was naturally in abundance around them when they were hungry.

Some skeptics may say that the life expectancy of the average prehistoric human was actually quite short, throwing doubt on the health benefits of our early ancestors' ways of living.

However, their life spans were no doubt affected by other circumstances rare in our modern lives, such as death by trauma or injury. Moreover, they lived in a lawless world and may have fought vicious battles against neighboring tribes and groups—and sometimes against each other.

Also, our prehistoric brethren were not at the top of the food chain; they were themselves hunted by large predators and did not always enjoy the constant abundance of food that we have today. Being fat and slow meant an easy, tasty meal for others!

They lived a much harsher and more violent life than modern humans, and died for many reasons beyond the scope of nutrition. Had they had constant access to readily available foods, and not suffered so many survival-related stresses, fewer would have died at an early age. Let's face it, a badly sprained ankle or broken arm could have meant death for our prehistoric ancestors. Indeed, in ideal circumstances, many prehistoric humans may have lived far longer—possibly longer than we do today.

The human body is, in fact, so resilient that it has contingency plans even when little or no food is available. Remember that periodic fasting (I will discuss this in great detail later in the book) would likely have been a part of pre-historic men/women's everyday lives. They would not have had access to a grocery store and been able to eat a bag of potato chips at midnight.

Having access to food at all times is a very recent modern phenomenon. Throw in the availability of highly processed food products, combined with a lack of exercise, and what you have is today's obesity problem. In short, understanding what makes us sick and unhealthy today requires us to take a look back in our history to see what made us thrive in order to be here today.

3

The Five Key Principles of *The Simple Life Healthy Lifestyle Plan*

It's important to strive for what is *realistic* rather than *idealistic*. In this spirit, *The Simple Life Healthy Lifestyle Plan* follows five truth-based, real-world principles designed to keep you on track. These form the practical foundation of *The Simple Life* concept as a whole, not just regarding health:

1. Knowledge is power

2. Avoid extremes

3. Keep it simple

4. Something is better than nothing

5. Take action today and every day

PRINCIPLE 1: KNOWLEDGE IS POWER

As you read this material, you may wonder why I have taken the time to go over *why* to do things and not just *what* to do. Well, it's because changing your life for the better, long-term, is not about fads or quick fixes. Moreover, I have a simple philosophy when it comes to health: *Knowledge is power.* With correct, in-depth information, you will see that nutrition and healthy living are simple to maintain.

But what is not simple is trying to change decades of bad health decisions based on bad information. Almost every day, another article or news program promotes a means to be healthy, yet most of the information is just flat-out wrong, often dangerous, and sometimes a bit of both.

Following advice you don't fully understand rarely results in success. Instead, new habits are most effective when you know *why* you are doing something. Otherwise, you're likely to be swayed by the next fad "miracle" diet or 10-minute workout program that comes along, without really understanding how it works (or more likely, that it doesn't).

Fad diets are often shrouded in vague pseudo-science and cheesy ads; I want you to have the truth about what you are eating and an understanding of the basics of exercise.

PRINCIPLE 2: AVOID EXTREMES

It's time to stop the fad madness!

Anytime I hear a phrase like "flat abs in just minutes a day!" or "lose five (or 10 or 12) pounds by the weekend!" I get really ticked off. Why? Because extreme claims may sound appealing, but they don't work. Once again, John Q. Public is the one to pay the price. While less sexy, a slow-and-steady healthy lifestyle approach, day after day, week after week, delivers true health and wellness—year after year!

Here's the bottom line: Any so-called health program that has you eating only one kind of "miracle" food (papaya and cabbage soup all day?), nuking something pre-packaged in a cardboard box for dinner, or paying for an expensive and complex piece of exercise equipment that an aging TV star favors *is to be avoided*. If it seems odd and sounds ridiculous, *it is*.

Extreme diet and exercise programs don't work in the long term!

Nevertheless, just like everyone else, I have fallen victim to numerous eating and exercise fads.

One of the most vivid memories I have on the topic is of a younger version of myself waking up two or three times a night with a friend to do hundreds of push-ups, sit-ups, pull-ups and other exercises, in addition to eating thousands of additional calories our bodies could never process. It sounded like a good idea at the time, but the results begged to differ—we just ended up fat and tired!

From such experiences I have learned a very important lesson: A fad is merely a fad for a reason, and diet and exercise fads have no basis in the continued pursuit of genuine health. Their main focus is to sell you something short-term. The purveyors of such works-for-the-moment "cures" don't care if their product or system works for the long term or not. When the diet-trick-of-the-month doesn't work, or stops working, guess who's ready to sell you the next miracle product?

But removing symptoms of poor health (such as excess fat) for a limited period of time does not cut to the real concern—the need to better care for our individual health statuses! Avoiding extremes is an important part of getting there.

PRINCIPLE 3: KEEP IT SIMPLE

Eating should be simple. If you pick up a food product in a grocery store and it contains ingredients you can't pronounce, or a list of ingredients so long that it takes up an entire side of the container, it's probably a bad choice. Plus, I'm pretty sure it wouldn't be recognized as food by our prehistoric ancestors.

As a culture, we have turned our concepts of eating and exercise into a confusing and overwhelming selection of products, regulations and fad diets. The government's involvement in the creation of nutritional guidelines shows how far we've drifted away from the basics of proper health and nutrition.

Against this backdrop of confusion, Americans spend more time worrying about how, when and what to eat than do the people of any other country. Did you know the average supermarket is 48,745 square feet in size and contains nearly 50,000 items? If you bought one item each day, it would take you over 125 years to sample all of them. No wonder we're confused about what to eat!

You don't need to understand biochemistry or be a nutritionist to feel good and be healthy. This book will cover a lot of in-depth information. However, it will be as user-friendly as possible.

Because, in reality, health is simple. Think of a primitive man or woman—they just had active lives, moved steadily throughout their days, and ate whole, natural foods.

PRINCIPLE 4: SOMETHING IS BETTER THAN NOTHING

At first, overhauling your entire lifestyle can seem daunting, especially if you have really let it get out of hand.

But here's a thought that always bears repeating: *Little changes and choices add up.* When it comes to doing nothing versus doing at least something, something is always the right choice. Think of it like dropping a dollar into a piggy bank every hour of the day for years and years...eventually you'd have a nice nest egg.

You can always do something! Instead of bemoaning your stressful, unhealthy life, answer this question: What would it take to make a healthier choice in this situation, at this exact moment? Even if it's only an incrementally better option, that little bit counts!

- Can't get to the gym? Do 10 minutes of push-ups, crunches and stretches in your living room. Even a few push-ups are better than none!

- No time to cook a healthy dinner? Skip the dollar-meal fast food takeout and pick up some pre-cooked chicken and a pre-made salad at the grocery store.

- Missed breakfast? Eat some nuts and a banana in your car on the way to work (kept there for just this purpose!)

- Sit at a desk all day with an aching back? Make it a point to stand up and move around each hour—even if only for two or three minutes!

- Exhausted and haven't seen your kids all day? Turn off the TV and catch up together on a brisk walk around the neighborhood (yes, they may complain, but try it anyway!)

When circumstances aren't ideal, don't assume you have no control. You always do. So instead of feeling bad that you can't do *everything*, do something!

PRINCIPLE 5: TAKE ACTION TODAY AND EVERY DAY

Look, America is full of people who *want* to be lean and strong and look good in a bathing suit. But, statistically, very few of us *are*. So what's the difference between those that wish and those that win?

Here's the simplest answer: Fit people take action, today and every day. Their lives are an answer to the question: What's it going to take to stay healthy today?

Maybe that means getting up a bit earlier to get to the gym. Maybe it means having a kitchen that doesn't get cleaned right away in order to make time for an exercise video while the kids nap. Maybe it means making a bagged lunch on Sunday night so that Monday's midday meal is healthy and inexpensive. Fit people think like this and take action, today and every day. Small choices add up to a lifestyle that dictates long-term success. That's the real-world truth.

So, what's it going to take for you to be fit and healthy today? Every day? This ties into Principle 4: **Something is Better Than Nothing**. If you can't get to the gym today, do some push-ups in your living room… today. Don't let not getting to the gym be an excuse for doing nothing. Always ask, if I can't do the ideal, what else can I do?

No time for a full workout today? How about taking the stairs instead of the elevator at every opportunity this week?

If you hurt your knee and can't run, what else can you do? Besides knee-friendly swimming and cycling, you could do a few bicep curls and ab exercises in your living room while watching the news. It won't make you an athlete, but it will help maintain fitness momentum.

Life gets hard, and healthy choices are sometimes inconvenient. Want to be lean and healthy? The secret is to make the right choices, slowly and surely, today and every day. Today's choices matter, and are under your control, every day.

That's the hard truth. But the good news is, once it's a habit it gets easy. Taking action is always the key.

Addressing Today's Common Health Myths

Many Americans have, unfortunately, been left with an inadequate working knowledge of how best to preserve their health, hence my Principle 1: **Knowledge is Power**.

Learning the truth about fat, obesity and exercise has changed my life, as well as my relationship with food. I know that this knowledge will have a profound effect on your life too!

Perhaps you, too, have been taught to believe some of the following falsehoods:

Myth #1: Eat as little fat as possible. Food choices should have the fat removed, even if it means substituting chemicals in its place.

Myth #2: Animal protein is bad for you. It causes heart disease, it raises your cholesterol, and it makes you fat (because it *contains* fat). Choose lean meat over other fat-filled meat.

Myth #3: You must exercise more to lose weight, because exercise is more important than diet.

Myth #4: Eat six to eleven servings of carbohydrates per day. And as long as the source of the carbohydrates is low-fat, it's okay.

This last falsehood was especially perpetuated for many years by the old USDA Food Pyramid, which outlined recommended eating habits for the American public. The Food Pyramid has recently changed to the updated MyPlate federal nutrition guidelines. Nevertheless, these old carb-dominant misconceptions unfortunately remain pervasive—and erroneous—beliefs to this day.

Below is an excerpt from the book *Good Calories, Bad Calories*, written by Gary Taubes, the only print journalist to win three Science in Society Journalism awards from the National Association of Science Writers. I don't agree with everything Taubes promotes, but I do agree with the majority of his groundbreaking conclusions in nutrition and science. Here are his words:

Throughout this research, I tried to follow the facts wherever they led. In writing the book, I have tried to let the science and the evidence speak for themselves. When I began my research, I had no idea that I would come to believe that obesity is not caused by eating too much, or that exercise is not a means of prevention. Nor did I believe that diseases such as cancer and Alzheimer's could possibly be caused by the consumption of refined carbohydrates and sugars. I had no idea that I would find the quality of the research on nutrition, obesity, and chronic disease to be so inadequate; that so much of the conventional wisdom would be founded on so little substantial evidence; and that, once it was, the researchers and the public-health authorities who funded the research would no longer see any reason to challenge this conventional wisdom and so to test its validity.

As I emerge from this research, though, certain conclusions seem inescapable to me, based on the existing knowledge:

1. Dietary fat, whether saturated or not, is not a cause of obesity, heart disease, or any other chronic disease of civilization.

2. The problem is the carbohydrates in the diet, their effect on insulin secretion, and thus the hormonal regulation of homeostasis—the entire harmonic ensemble of the human body. The more easily digestible and refined the carbohydrates, the greater the effect on our health, weight, and wellbeing.

3. Sugars—sucrose and high-fructose corn syrup specifically—are particularly harmful, probably because the combination of fructose and glucose simultaneously elevates insulin levels while overloading the liver with carbohydrates.

4. Through their direct effect on insulin and blood sugar, refined carbohydrates, starches, and sugars are the dietary cause of coronary heart disease and diabetes. They are the most likely dietary causes of cancer, Alzheimer's disease, and the other chronic diseases of civilization.

5. Obesity is a disorder of excess fat accumulation, not overeating, and not sedentary behavior.

6. Consuming excess calories does not cause us to grow

fatter, any more than it causes a child to grow taller. Expending more energy than we consume does not lead to long-term weight loss; it leads to hunger.

7. Fattening and obesity are caused by an imbalance—a disequilibrium—in the hormonal regulation of adipose tissue and fat metabolism. Fat synthesis and storage exceed the mobilization of fat from the adipose tissue and its subsequent oxidation. We become leaner when the hormonal regulation of the fat tissue reverses this balance.

8. Insulin is the primary regulator of fat storage. When insulin levels are elevated—either chronically or after a meal—we accumulate fat in our fat tissue. When insulin levels fall, we release fat from our fat tissue and use it for fuel.

9. By stimulating insulin secretion, carbohydrates make us fat and ultimately cause obesity. The fewer carbohydrates we consume, the leaner we will be.

10. By driving fat accumulation, carbohydrates also increase hunger and decrease the amount of energy we expend in metabolism and physical activity.

You may now be curious as to why so many of Taubes' ideas run contrary to the weight loss how-to's commonly promoted by morning television and newsstand magazines.

We'll debunk these macronutrient myths in detail throughout this book. But first, what exactly is a macronutrient?

Macronutrients are chemical compounds that, when eaten, provide fuel (energy) to your body. The three major categories of macronutrients are *carbohydrates, fats* and *proteins*. Each will be discussed in detail in this book.

I've called them macronutrient myths because, as you've seen, most of what we've been taught about nutrition—from magazines, government health initiatives, in school, and certainly from the food industry—is likely just plain wrong.

Experts, scientific literature, schools and our government all play influential roles in what we perceive healthy living to mean. However, much of this previously accepted information may be proven incorrect as new research and thinking emerges, and as older, previously repressed or forgotten research is revealed.

To start, let's consider why almost all of us need a huge dietary overhaul.

REVERSING THE WESTERN DIET

Of particular relevance to our journey together will be your understanding of what most Americans eat today: the so-called *Western Diet*. You have, of course, likely heard this term many times, but you may not understand what it actually entails. The Western Diet is typically eaten in developed (and some developing) countries throughout the world. It is heavily weighted toward processed foods, factory-farmed meat, unhealthy fats and oils, sugars, and refined grains. Fruits, vegetables and unprocessed, fresh foods of any type are largely missing.

Populations who eat a standard Western Diet tend to suffer from high rates of obesity, type 2 diabetes and cardiovascular disease. Some research indicates that more than a third of all cancers (I argue that it's closer to half) can be linked to this way of eating.

It gets worse. Industrially produced foods prevalent in the developed world frequently contain unnatural chemicals and hormones. Recent research from the Cincinnati Children's Hospital

Medical Center has shown that young girls are starting to undergo puberty earlier—some as young as seven or eight years old. These chemical endocrine disruptors are implicated in other metabolic disorders involving thyroid dysfunction, mood impairment and more.

Does the Western Diet sound like your way of eating? I know it used to be mine. How did we learn to eat this way? From our schools, popular cookbooks, government food recommendations or our family? Perhaps it was a bit of each. What's certain is that the typical Western Diet leads to impaired health and an earlier demise than do the eating habits of poorer, less developed countries, where food is still fresh, clean and unprocessed.

Thanks to medical advances, we live longer than we used to. But what is the benefit of these added years if they are spent in and out of hospitals with chronic diet-related diseases or while not feeling well? Who wants to be wasting away for years with cancer due to a condition caused by the Western Diet? I know I don't!

Our advances in medicine, health care and science are exciting, but relying on them to prolong an unhealthy life is not the answer. If an individual lives longer than his forebears, yet is sick and miserable, it's no blessing for him or his family and community!

But there is good news. Years of research now indicate that the effects of the Western Diet can, for the most part, be reversed. Studies have shown that people who have abandoned the Western Diet for a more traditional and natural diet will regain health and reduce their chances of suffering from the usual Western Diet-induced chronic diseases.

To solve this problem, you'll need to understand the *right* way to eat carbohydrates, fats and proteins.

Why It Takes Guts to Be Healthy

HOW BACTERIA RULE YOUR INTESTINES AND YOUR LIFE

People are usually shocked when I start discussing gut bacteria before I even mention a word about exercise or macronutrients (carbs, proteins and fats). I can't make it any simpler than this: As far as health goes, it all starts in your gut! Those trillions of microbes in our guts keep us alive—without them we die, plain and simple. You treat them unkindly, and they will return the favor. The healthier your gut, the healthier *you* are. No magic abs machine, or other health fad of the moment, will compare to this.

Your gastrointestinal tract is considered one of the most complex microbial ecosystems in the world. The microbes in your gut not only affect your digestion, but your entire health. It is estimated that nearly 100 trillion fungi, bacteria, viruses and other microorganisms compose your body's micro-flora. You have 10-to-1 bacteria to cells in your body. Basically, humans are living bacteria, and without them our species would cease to exist. To say that this relationship between bacteria and the human host is essential, but yet greatly misunderstood by most, is an understatement.

According to Dr. Natasha Campell-McBride, M.D., gut microflora can be divided into three groups:

1. Essential or beneficial flora. This is the most important group and the most numerous in a healthy individual. These bacteria are often referred to as our indigenous friendly bacteria.

2. Opportunistic flora. This is a large group of various microbes. There are around 500 known various species of microbes that can be found in the human gut (and this number is increasing all the time). In a healthy person, their numbers are usually limited and tightly controlled by the beneficial flora. If any one of these microbes becomes out of balance, it can cause a host of health problems.

3. Transitional flora. These are various microbes that we daily swallow with food and liquids. When we are healthy and the gut is well protected by beneficial bacteria, this group of microbes will pass through our digestive system without causing harm. But if our gut flora is out of balance, this group of microbes can cause disease. Basically, on a daily basis we are exposed to good, bad and transitional bacteria, and our overall gut health determines whether these microbes will promote good or bad health. There is an ebb and flow constantly going on in your gut micro-flora. The general rule is, our gut, when functioning properly, is 85% good bacteria and 15% bad bacteria.

So why would we have an estimated 15% of what is considered to be harmful microbes in our gut, you may ask? The good and bad bacteria keep each other in check so one will not override the other and cause an imbalance. There is a complex language being spoken in your gut, where various chemicals attach to receptor sites on these microbes, letting each side know when it's time to create or destroy one or the other to keep everything working properly. If this check system was not in place, you could literally be taken over by a group, or groups, of beneficial or harmful bacteria.

What Is Leaky Gut Syndrome and How Does It Impact Your Health?

Leaky gut syndrome (LGS) is a condition that happens when gaps develop between the cells (enterocytes) that line your intestinal wall. These tiny gaps allow substances, such as undigested food, harmful proteins, bacteria, viruses, yeast and metabolic wastes, to enter into your bloodstream. These harmful substances should be confined to your digestive tract in order to maintain proper digestion and health.

Once the integrity of your intestinal lining is compromised (damaged cells called microvilli become unable to do their job properly), this causes a flow of harmful substances to leak into your bloodstream. You then also become unable to process and utilize the nutrients and enzymes that are vital for proper digestion. The end result is that your body experiences harmful inflammation, often referred to as chronic inflammation. Your body then goes into attack mode trying to kill or eradicate these harmful substances. This is what is generally called the autoimmune response. Basically, your immune system is attacking itself.

Leaky gut syndrome is often associated with inflammatory bowel diseases like ulcerative colitis, Crohn's or celiac disease, along with many other autoimmune diseases.

In addition to the above, people who suffer from leaky gut

syndrome will often experience some, or many, of the common ailments below:

- Food allergies

- Seasonal allergies

- Asthma

- Sore, swollen joints

- Frequent stomach aches

- Diarrhea, followed by constipation (or vice versa)

- Arthritis

- Eczema

- Frequent heartburn

- Frequent colds

- Frequent sinus/upper respiratory infections

- Chronic fatigue

- Frequent headaches/migraines

- Gas/bloating/cramps

- Chronic or frequent yeast infections

There are many more health conditions related to LGS, but these are the most common ones I've seen when working with clients.

In my case, I experienced terrible seasonal allergies from a very young age, and numerous visits to doctors and specialists could not solve this issue. I thought I was doomed to suffer from debilitating allergies for the remainder of my life. But once I changed to what I now like to call my *Simple Life Diet* (because it helps make my life much easier), my allergies almost completely disappeared. I had probably been suffering from LGS for decades and didn't even know it.

I know I'm not alone in this experience, as I have worked with thousands of clients and sold tens of thousands of books on the subject of health.

Happy Gut, Happy Brain

Recently, there has been a great deal learned about how our brains are directly affected by the health of our gut and the bacteria contained within. Our brains are connected to our guts via the *vagus nerve*, which is a large, complex nerve that runs throughout the body from the brain to the gut. As a matter of fact, it is now well established that the vagus nerve is the primary route your gut bacteria use to transmit information to your brain.

Today researchers are discovering that your mental health is very much dependent on the microbes in your gut. Recently *The Scientific American* reported:

> *Scientists are increasingly convinced that the vast assemblage of microfauna in our intestines may have a major impact on our state of mind. The gut-brain axis seems to be bidirectional—the brain acts on gastrointestinal and immune functions that help to shape the gut's microbial makeup, and gut microbes make neuroactive compounds, including neurotransmitters and metabolites that also act on the brain.*

In addition, an article published in the June 2013 issue of *Biological Psychiatry* suggests that even severe and chronic mental health problems, including post-traumatic stress disorder (PTSD), might be eliminated through the use of certain probiotics (healthy bacteria found in our guts).

One of the factors that amazes most individuals who implement my *Simple Life Health* philosophy, is how much better their cognitive function becomes (intellectual process by which one becomes aware of, perceives or comprehends ideas).

Simply, healthy gut = healthy brain!

What to Avoid When Trying to Maintain a Healthy Gut

- Unnecessary use, or overuse, of antibiotics

- Long-term use of pharmaceutical drugs

- Environmental exposure to harmful chemicals

- Eating conventionally raised meat—80% of all antibiotics used in the United States are fed or administered to animals raised in Confined Animal Feeding Operations (CAFOs)

- Consuming processed foods

- Consuming foods high in fructose, sugar or artificial sweeteners

- Eating fruits and vegetables grown using chemical herbicides and pesticides

- Chlorinated and/or fluoridated water

- Regularly using antibacterial soaps

How to Reseed and Maintain Your Gut Health

Reseeding your gut with beneficial bacteria is essential for maintaining proper balance. Beneficial bacteria help keep pathogenic microbes and fungi in check, preventing them from taking over.

In addition to avoiding the above, I recommend below four ways to help restore and maintain a healthy gut. I want to emphasize this: It takes time for you to rebuild your gut bacteria; it doesn't happen overnight. It took about two years for my gut to heal and for my seasonal allergies to all but disappear. For some this may happen quicker, but on average it will take several months.

1. Get dirty.

Get outside—the soil, and outdoor environment, is teeming with beneficial bacteria.

Use less soap. That's right, you heard me right—we chronically over clean ourselves. Your body is coated with all kinds of friendly microbes. These friendly microbes not only coat your skin, offering a layer of protection, but make their way inside you. Part of your initial gut flora is seeded by absorbing, via your skin, beneficial microbes when you are born and pass through your mother's vaginal canal.

2. Consume fermented foods and drinks.

- Kefir (organic)

- Pickles

- Cabbage

- Carrots

- Squash

- Kombucha

3. Consume prebiotics.

Prebiotics are non-digestible foods that help good bacteria grow and flourish. To get your dose of prebiotics, consume foods high in fiber primarily in the form of fruits, nuts and vegetables.

4. Take probiotic supplements.

Probiotics provide the human gut with multiple supportive functions. Often referred to as beneficial bacteria, these microorganisms help to digest lactose and protein, regulate bowel motility, and keep the GI tract functioning optimally.

I carry a probiotic that I have used for years to improve my and my clients' gut health on my website: **www.thesimplelifenow.com**.

6

Why Are We Addicted to Refined Carbohydrates?

CARBOHYDRATES DEFINED

What exactly is a carbohydrate? Sugars, starches and fibers are all considered to be dietary carbohydrates, since they have similar chemical structures. More specifically, they are all made up of a collection of carbon, hydrogen and oxygen molecules, with a two-to-one ratio of hydrogen to oxygen.

Carbohydrates are naturally occurring, organic substances. According to some nutrition scientists, they are essential for life. The brain and central nervous system can function on a continuous supply of carbohydrate-derived glucose, which is the principal circulating sugar in the blood and the body's major energy source when dietary carbohydrates are plentiful.

The amount of carbohydrates you consume affects the fuel your body uses and the way it stores fat. In a nutshell, if you eat too many carbohydrates, the excess amount will often be stored as fat. Too few, and your body will cannibalize your muscles for nutrition.

If you're reading this book, it's a safe bet you'd like to burn fat, right? Good news: With the right diet, the human body can also derive fuel from ketones, which are the metabolic energy units of fat metabolism. These provide a steady source of energy over a long period of time. The secret is to eat the right kinds of carbs in the right amounts. That's what we'll discuss in this section.

These concepts will be returned to and discussed in depth throughout this book. For now, note that eliminating excess carbohydrates—and particularly sugar and white flour-based products—is the key to a successful fitness and weight loss program.

Here's the carb low-down you'll need to maximize fat loss:

Empty Carbohydrates are carbohydrate-based foods that are highly processed, usually containing mainly sugar, white flour and vitality-sapping additives and chemicals. They only provide calories and contain very little (or no) nutritional value. Translation: Your waistline increases while your energy decreases.

Refined Carbohydrates (a type of empty carb) are produced when carbohydrate-rich plants are processed in a way that strips away everything but the most quickly digestible components (which are starches and/or sugars).

This unnatural technique removes healthy components, such as vitamins, and concentrates the carbohydrates. Your body then processes them very rapidly, usually causing an unhealthy spike in blood sugar.

Refined and highly processed carbohydrates—such as processed (usually white) breads, pastas, packaged oatmeal and processed cereals—are digested rapidly. This can result in a concurrently rapid rise in blood sugar and a slow rise in your pant size.

Health-Giving Carbohydrates are natural carbohydrate-based foods that contain vitamins and minerals that our bodies need for optimal health. Most of the carbohydrates you eat should come from the following health-giving sources: fruits, vegetables and nuts. To clarify, your primary carbohydrate source should come from vegetables, with nuts and fruits scattered in. Most people over consume fruits in their path to lose weight, but the fact is there is not one nutrient you cannot get from vegetables that is contained in fruit. People will often eat handfuls of nuts daily thinking that's the way to go. Yes, nuts are a nutritious food, but they contain a high Omega 6-to-Omega 3 ratio and should be moderately consumed.

These foods help control your blood sugar, energy and insulin (an important regulatory hormone; we'll discuss insulin in detail as we continue). They also help keep you lean and fit. Not surprisingly, these are the kinds of carbs at the core of *The Simple Life Healthy Lifestyle Plan.*

SUGAR

The truth about common table sugar is not so sweet: It is **not** a source of health-supporting vitamins, fiber or minerals, but instead contains several chemicals that are not conducive to health. This is why it is sometimes called a source of empty calories.

Indeed, table sugar has no nutritional value whatsoever. Consuming sugar actually robs your body of vitamins, minerals, and even enzymes, which are sacrificed for its metabolism. Sadly, sugary foods often displace more healthful foods, such as fruits and vegetables, in our diets. Thus people who eat sugar-rich diets get less calcium, fiber, zinc, iron and magnesium, as well as vitamins A, C and E amongst other nutrients.

Sugar, Our Drug of Choice?

You can, in fact, become addicted to table (refined) sugar, as recent research indicates. Yes, that's right: Refined sugar can be considered an addictive drug.

Researchers of sugar addiction note that removing sugar from your diet can induce drug withdrawal-like symptoms as excruciating and serious as those associated with alcohol withdrawal. These may include tremors, flu-like symptoms, headaches and mood swings. A 2002 Princeton University study conducted on rats demonstrated that sugar could be as addictive as heroin.

Neuroscientist Bart Hoebel, who led the Princeton study, noted that sugar triggers production of the brain's natural opioids (morphine-like chemicals that dull pain). "We think that is a key to the addiction process," he said. "The brain is getting addicted to its own opioids as it would to morphine or heroin. Drugs give a bigger effect, but it is essentially the same process."

"The implication is that some animals, and some people, can become overly dependent on sweet food, particularly if they periodically stop eating and then binge," Hoebel continued. "This may relate to eating disorders such as bulimia."

Below are five reasons sugar is considered by some researchers to be an addictive substance:

1. Symptoms similar to withdrawal seem to occur when sugar consumption ceases or is rapidly reduced.

2. Neurotransmitters in the brain are impacted in the same manner as when alcohol and hard drugs, like cocaine, are abused.

3. With continued use, tolerance occurs and sugar consumption must be increased to achieve the same experience.

4. Sugar is often eaten compulsively, despite negative consequences or a desire to stop.

5. Sugar consumption (for example, drinking soda) is required for everyday functioning.

How Sugar Saps Your Health

Further destructive effects of sugar include damaging, altering and disrupting the proper functioning of the nervous system, endocrine (glandular and hormonal) system, metabolic (energy and fat-burning) system, cardiovascular system, gastrointestinal system and immune (disease-fighting) system, as well as primary organs like the liver, kidneys, colon and pancreas. The American Diabetes Association considers the consumption of sugar to be one of the three major causes of degenerative disease in America. Sugar is so destructive that it can probably be linked to just about any harmful health condition you can think of.

While the entirety of sugar's negative health impacts is beyond the scope of this discussion, what follows are some of the most common concerns:

- Hormone imbalance

- Addiction

- Depression

- Mood swings

- Chronic fatigue

- Irritability

- Obesity

- Hyperactivity

- Mineral depletion

- Cancer

- Anxiety

- Panic attacks

- Chromium deficiency

- Depletion of the adrenal glands

- Type 2 diabetes

- Hypoglycemia

- Immune system problems

- Obesity

- High cholesterol

- Anti-social behaviors such as those found in crime and delinquency

- Anger control issues

- Insomnia

- Aggression

- Neurotransmitter deficiencies

- High blood pressure

- Heart disease

- Asthma

- Pre-menstrual syndrome (PMS)

- Obsessive-compulsive disorder (OCD)

- Attention deficit disorder (ADD)

- Binge eating

The American Sugar Overload

It is estimated that the average American consumes 175 pounds of sugar per year, and that number is going up. That's approximately 46 teaspoons of sugar per day, or close to 20 percent of our overall caloric intake! In contrast, in the late 1800s average sugar consumption was said to be around five pounds per person per year—and in that era, cardiovascular disease and cancer were nearly unheard of.

It is generally accepted that you should not consume more than eight teaspoons of sugar per day. This includes refined sugars as well as naturally occurring sugars in sweet-tasting whole foods (such as fruits).

To truly grasp the actual amount of sugar the average American consumes per day, pour 46 teaspoons of sugar into a bowl and see how much sugar this really is. Consuming that much sugar in one sitting would make you, at the very least, quite ill, or even worse, could induce a life-threatening coma!

As a matter of fact, one teaspoon of sugar equals around four to five grams. A 12-ounce can of Coke has 39 grams of sugar— nearly 10 teaspoons! This is more than the total recommended sugar consumption for an *entire* day.

Our Daily Sugar, Broken Down

The average American's daily sugar intake might play out like this:

Breakfast: 1.5 cups cereal, 1 cup of juice, 1 cup of milk
= 10 tsp sugar

Snack: 2 toaster pastries and 1 can of soft drink
= 15 tsp sugar

Lunch: 1 sandwich, 1 granola bar, 1 cup apple juice
= 7 tsp sugar

Snack: 1 serving applesauce, 1 cup Gatorade = 7 tsp sugar

Dinner: salad with dressing, 1 potato, pork chops, 2 cookies
= 6 tsp sugar

TOTAL = 45 teaspoons of sugar (180 grams)

For many, this list seems like a fairly healthy menu. But with 45 teaspoons of sugar, healthy it is not.

The typical American diet is completely out of balance. How does your daily diet compare to the above? Is it better or worse? The bottom line is this: Eat less than eight teaspoons of sugar per day—from all sources—to maximize weight loss and health.

To ensure you stay below the eight-teaspoon limit, diligently read the labels of all food products you purchase. The amount of sugar in a serving will be listed on the package. You may find many seemingly healthy foods are actually loaded with sugar. For example, some fruit juices can contain up to 50 grams (10 to 12 teaspoons!) of sugar in one 8-ounce serving.

Sugar and Carbohydrate Intolerance

Have you ever said something like, "If I just look at a doughnut, I gain weight"? Do you feel physically uncomfortable after eating sugar- or carb-rich foods? If so, you may have an intolerance to certain foods.

Sugar Intolerance: People who are intolerant to sugar generally gain weight rapidly if they consume sugary foods.

Different types of sugars are chemically processed in the body by different types of enzymes. For example, the enzyme sucrase breaks down the sugar sucrose; the enzyme lactase breaks down lactose. You may develop a sugar intolerance if you become deficient in any enzyme that is required to process any specific sugar. Causes of this condition include normal aging and genetic origins.

Symptoms of sugar intolerance include nervousness, anxiety, heart palpations and arrhythmias, indigestion accompanied by bloating and flatulence, fatigue, joint pain, forgetfulness and confusion. It has also been associated with insulin resistance, type 2 diabetes and rapid weight gain.

Carbohydrate Intolerance: It is also possible to be carbohydrate intolerant. This occurs when the small intestine is unable to completely process carbs (including sugars and starches) into a source of energy for the body.

This is also usually due to deficiency of a particular digestive enzyme. No treatment exists for this problem other than the dietary control of symptoms (i.e., choosing not to eat carbs). Carbohydrate intolerance may also be caused by temporary intestinal diseases. In such cases, it usually disappears when the underlying condition is successfully treated.

Carbohydrate intolerance is similar to sugar intolerance, since carbohydrates either start as simple sugars (monosaccharides) or are broken down into simple sugars during digestion. Symptoms of carbohydrate intolerance include diarrhea, abdominal distention and flatulence.

HIGH BLOOD SUGAR, HIGH FAT STORAGE: THE INSULIN CONNECTION

We'll now hone in on an incredibly important concept at the heart of your health and weight-loss success: how the hormone insulin influences weight loss (or gain!), and why carb consumption is the key to this regulation.

You want to be lean and healthy? You need to understand insulin; period.

Simple Life Health Point: The presence of sugar in the blood and the subsequent release of the hormone insulin play important roles in fat storage and weight gain. You must understand insulin's influence to succeed in your weight-loss goals!

What is Insulin?

Insulin, in brief, is a hormone secreted by the pancreas that serves to coordinate and regulate the storage and use of nutrients and the maintenance of homeostasis (a healthy physiological balance) in your body. Stated another way, it ensures you have healthy blood sugar levels and prevents sugar-induced imbalances.

Insulin is a very powerful hormone—the most powerful when it comes to fat storage. The bottom line: If you control your insulin levels through quality food choices, you will see remarkable changes in your physical appearance and your mental well-being. It doesn't get simpler than that.

How Insulin Works

Here's how insulin keeps your health in check: When your blood sugar levels increase rapidly, or are continuously heightened because you've eaten a lot of sugars or refined carbohydrates (*empty* carbs), your body produces insulin. Insulin "mops up" the sugars and stores them in the most accessible energy storage option your body has: fat tissue.

Without insulin, you could literally get sick or die from drastic blood sugar fluctuations (a problem at the core of diabetes.) Simply put, insulin's job is to save your life.

Let's review: You eat a sugary food -> you have too much sugar in your blood -> your body releases insulin -> the insulin stores the excess sugar as fat -> your blood sugar levels return to normal.

Our prehistoric brethren would not have needed this life-saving response very frequently since they didn't eat many sweet foods. However, in our convenience-food world, we are overtaxed by sugar-laden snacks. Your body wants you to give it a break!

But remember, sugar doesn't just come from candies and cakes. Refined carbohydrates, such as those present in white flour-based foods, are broken down into simple sugars as you eat and digest them. That's right: Eating white bread is kind of like eating candy, at least as far as your fat-storing hormones are concerned.

To get lean and healthy, ditch the white bread and pasta and eat the same high-quality, real foods your ancestors would have, like fresh vegetables and organic meats. At the core of *The Simple Life Healthy Lifestyle Plan* is choosing far fewer refined carbs and more healthy fats and proteins; period. **In fact, if you did nothing but drop white flour-based and sugar-filled foods from your life, you would already have taken a huge step toward better health.**

Of course, refraining from sweetened, white flour pseudo-foods does not mean banishing all carbs entirely from your diet. I firmly believe in avoiding extremes. Instead of total elimination, relegate refined sugar and white flour-based products to occasional treat status only!

But, I will tell you from personal experience and working with thousands of clients, once you banish these highly processed carbs and sugars from your diet, your body is not going to like it when you try to re-introduce these foreign foods back into your diet...even as an occasional treat.

Insulin's Powerful Influence

Let's review the impact that a sugar-driven insulin surge has on your body:

1. It leads to carb crashes. Insulin encourages your body to use more carbohydrates, and less fat, as fuel. This leads to detrimental energy crashes and carb cravings.

In your body, refined carbohydrates are like kindling: They burn fast and hot, are used up quickly, and must be continually replenished to produce energy. Energy from refined carbs is short-lived just as kindling for a fire is quickly exhausted. This is why a sugary breakfast of cold cereal and orange juice is quickly burned off, providing a temporary surge of energy followed by a mid-morning slump.

This renewed hunger and fatigue leads to another carbohydrate-based snack, and another temporary elevation in energy, followed by the inevitable fall. This cycle continues all throughout the day, with concomitant rises and falls in insulin levels. You feel exhausted and your pants slowly get tighter.

If the problem is continuous, you may never get rid of the pounds and you'll be chronically exhausted. Does this sound like your story?

2. It encourages fat storage. Insulin converts almost half of your dietary carbohydrates to fat. So if you want to burn away the pounds (i.e., use more stored fat for energy), you must discourage the release of insulin in your body.

3. It causes hunger, which often leads to overeating. If you eat a meal that is high in carbohydrates, your blood sugar will tend to increase rapidly. Therefore, insulin levels concurrently rise in order to stabilize your blood sugar levels (i.e., bring them back down to homeostasis). This decrease in blood sugar then stimulates hunger, often soon after a meal, and perpetuates the vicious cycle described in the first point above.

4. It hinders helpful hormones. High insulin levels suppress the actions of important fat-burning, muscle-building hormones. These are *glucagon* (a hormone secreted by the pancreas that increases blood sugar levels) and *growth hormone.*

Glucagon promotes the burning of fat and sugar. Growth hormone is used for building new muscle mass and muscle development. So if you want to burn fat and sugar and build muscle, you will need to maintain high levels of both hormones by avoiding high insulin levels in your body.

How Glucagon Works

If we created an overly simplified version of how fat storage and fat burning work in the body, it would look something like this:

- You eat a lot of sugar/simple carbs -> your body releases **insulin** -> the sugar is stored as fat tissue -> your waistline increases

- You don't eat sugar/simple carbs -> your body releases **glucagon** -> your body burns fat for energy -> your waistline decreases

When sugar (and therefore insulin) is *not* present in the blood, the body begins to use fat as its energy source through a process known as gluconeogenesis. This process is activated by the hormone glucagon, a pancreatic hormone that works in opposition to insulin.

Glucagon stimulates an increase in blood sugar levels, opposing the sugar-decreasing actions of insulin. **But if you eat a sugary snack that stimulates it into action, insulin will hinder the release of glucagon.**

In this way, insulin prevents the use of fat as an energy source (i.e., it keeps you from burning fat and therefore prevents you from losing weight).

The Insulin Solution

How can you avoid insulin-related weight gain? Some of the most powerful actions you can take are as follows:

1. Eat fewer sugars and refined carbohydrates. This should be obvious by now!

2. Eat more fiber. Fiber-rich foods slow your body's insulin response. Insulin responses vary greatly from person to person. Generally, refined foods (such as pastries, white potatoes, white pastas, white rice or white breads) evoke a stronger and/or more rapid insulin reaction than unrefined carbohydrates (think sweet potatoes or yams). This is because refined carbohydrates have been stripped of their natural fiber and, in the case of grains, their oil-bearing germ during processing.

This dietary fiber would otherwise have minimized or slowed the body's carbohydrate/insulin response.

3. Or do both! Note that foods that contain simple sugars rarely contain fiber, so by avoiding sweet foods you usually kill two dietary birds with one stone. Remember, without fiber there is nothing to slow down the digestion of sugary foods. This leads to excessive insulin release (a.k.a. the dreaded insulin spike), which slows or stops the body from using fat as an energy source. In other words: processed sweet foods = less fat burning and less weight loss.

Of course, eating lots of fiber does not automatically lead to weight loss. But, generally speaking, aim to avoid sugary foods.

Dieter's Dilemma

Here's a frequent weight loss mistake: To lose weight, a dieter decides to have a light lunch. He or she then eats only a baked potato. This sounds reasonable when we use old theories on dieting (eating fewer calories and much less fat leads to weight loss), but if you want to lose fat, or if you are carbohydrate sensitive, then this is the wrong approach. Why? Because it's not the amount of calories, but the quality of calories you consume, that allows you to lose and maintain a healthy weight. (More on calories later.)

Making matters worse, our dieter will often wash down the potato with a sugary soda or sports drink (most of which contain 20 or more grams of sugar). Now we have the perfect storm: a fast-acting simple carbohydrate (the soda or sports drink) followed by a slower-acting complex carbohydrate (the potato).

The result? Blood sugar levels rise higher, over a longer period of time. This stimulates the release of more insulin, which stays in the blood for a sustained period and leads to increased fat storage.

Even today, the above example is looked upon by many as the perfect dieter's meal, just adding to more confusion. I have witnessed misguided dieters opt for this meal as part of an attempt at weight loss more times than I can count.

Remember: When you are trying to lose weight (fat), do not eat carbohydrates or simple sugars alone. This can often seem counterintuitive. For example, a dieter may eat one piece, several pieces, or even most of their calories in the form of sweet-tasting fruit, by itself.

While fruit is healthy, when eaten alone it is not ideal for weight loss. If weight loss is your goal, eat fruit (and especially very sweet types of fruit), with or immediately after a meal that contains digestion-slowing proteins, fats or fiber. This will dull your body's insulin response to the sugars and help you to store less fat.

Carbohydrates and Water Retention: A Real-Life Example

People who consume a disproportionate amount of refined carbohydrates almost always have a puffy look to them. As you can see from our discussion, this has to do with how their bodies use insulin and retain sodium (and therefore water). One example of this phenomenon in particular comes to mind.

Years ago, I knew a young woman who didn't give much consideration to her diet. She was in college and ate like she was in college, which means her diet was made up of many refined carbohydrates and a lot of fast food. She enjoyed frequent Mexican food splurges, and socialized over cocktails and other alcoholic drinks with friends. Sounds harmless, right? Sadly, it wasn't.

Fortunately, she was physically active. However, she did not realize her diet was a hindrance to good health, despite consistent workouts. Thus she experienced many diet-related health troubles such as fluctuations in weight, water retention, bloating, years of stomach issues and fatigue.

Many people today find themselves with similar symptoms, mostly because they eat way too many refined carbohydrates. For my friend, fluctuating weight loss or a weight gain of seven to ten pounds in a span of three to five days was a frequent occurrence.

Although the amount of food she ate each day stayed relatively constant, her symptoms were heightened when she ate mainly processed carbohydrates.

As we've discussed, bloating and water retention are symptomatic of high levels of blood-borne insulin and the retention of sodium. However, two medications, a CT scan, and one colonoscopy later, doctors still could not find out what was wrong with my young friend. So, with my help, she began to run her own experiment with a healthier, more balanced diet. Soon she didn't need her medications, or any more doctor visits, and she has maintained a consistent weight ever since. By recently fine-tuning her diet, she lost an additional 15 pounds and now weighs the same as she did in high school.

The only time she has stomach issues now is when she treats herself to a very occasional meal at a restaurant. This is not surprising, since typically the body will become accustomed to eating better, healthier foods and it will noticeably object when anything that is less than healthful is reintroduced.

If only her doctors had spent more time researching her nutritional habits and helping her to eat fewer carbs, she could have saved a lot of money, time and distress.

At this point you may be wondering what my formula was for diet change in the preceding story. Well, there was one thing that immediately stuck out to me when I analyzed my friend's diet. Specifically, she consumed almost no protein or healthy fats. Her everyday diet was comprised primarily of bagels, sugary and processed yogurt products, and granola bars. She would literally go days just eating those three items.

The amazing part is that she has a background in modern-day nutrition and thought she was eating a perfectly healthy diet! I would like to say that this type of belief is the exception, but sadly this is what I find is the case with many of the people with whom I work. They, too, eat mostly processed carbohydrates in the mistaken belief that they are eating a healthy diet, since this approach is promoted by many health and medical communities as the best way to avoid weight problems and illness.

But Don't We Need Carbs to Survive?

Today's health community often claims that "proper" amounts of carbs are necessary to thrive, since your body needs carbs in order to produce glucose. This is not the case, as your body has a backup system that uses amino acids (the building blocks of protein) and fats to form glucose. Thus, without any dietary carbs you will not waste away, and (barring outright starvation) your body will not cannibalize your muscles to fuel your body.

How does this backup system work? *Glycogen* is the storage form of carbohydrates in humans and animals and is found mainly in liver and muscle tissue. It is readily converted to glucose (a sugar), when required, to satisfy the body's energy needs.

In other words, after you have used all readily available blood glucose for your immediate energy needs, your body will turn to this stored glucose (glycogen) as a backup energy source. The human body typically packs about 400 grams (14 ounces) of glycogen into its liver and muscle cells.

Nevertheless, take note: I do not advocate eliminating *all* carbs from your diet. After all, vegetables contain carbohydrates and I recommend eating a lot of those!

THE RIGHT WAY TO EAT CARBS

Some people will experience a decrease in energy or more fatigue and sleep problems when strictly avoiding all carbohydrates. These folks must eat some carbohydrates, and if they are in the form of grains they must be properly prepared for optimum digestibility and in the appropriate quantities for their constitutions. What do I mean by this? And what about the gluten-free debate? I'll delve into the gluten issue at the end of this section.

Grains in their natural state—such as wheat or oatmeal—are not meant to be consumed by humans, or at the very least not long-term as your primary nutrition source. In this form they are seeds, which are meant to pass through mammalian digestive tracts and get deposited in a nice pile of fertilizer, ready to grow.

Grains in their natural forms contain many toxic proteins and other natural chemicals that actually harm your digestive system and cause numerous health problems (they are one of the primary causes of leaky gut syndrome).

I encourage you to greatly reduce your grain consumption and, for many, completely eliminate them (remember, you can get carbs and fiber from non-grain sources such as vegetables, nuts, and fruits.) When you do eat grains, or foods made of grains, they should be sprouted or soaked.

Sprouted grains have been released from their toxic protein-rich pods and are easier to digest. This is something you can easily do at home, although you can also buy sprouted grain products at natural food markets and even in many supermarkets (typically in the frozen foods section.) That being said, people with grain sensitivities can still suffer health issues from sprouted grains.

Soaking grains is something you can do at home to help break down whole-grain-based toxins. Soak brown rice or oatmeal (yes, this is raw grain) for 24 hours in filtered water mixed with a tablespoon of vinegar or lemon juice. This acid base will help break down the chemicals detrimental to your health. Then just rinse off the grains and cook as you normally would.

I give the above as an option, but I'm a firm believer in going completely grain-free for most people. During my decades of self-experimentation and working with clients, I have seen way too many benefits of removing all or most grains than to try and figure out which ones might not give you problems. If there is one exception, I would say it is white rice. I have found most people do not seem to have a negative reaction to this grain. Remember, though, white rice is a starchy carbohydrate and must be consumed in moderation to avoid insulin spikes and unwanted weight gain.

To Grain or Not to Grain

When it comes to consuming grains, it can get a little confusing. The Paleo Diet is well known for eliminating grains completely, as grains are considered one of the three most inflammatory foods. The other two are beans and dairy.

In some cases, when properly prepared, soaked for 24 hours, or sprouted, grains are considered acceptable by some groups. Others say no to grains; period.

Where do I land in the questionable grain universe? I feel that, due to their minimal nutritional content and the energy needed to digest them, they are not worth the effort to include in my or your diet. In addition, I feel that grains were never intended to be digested by humans as a primary food source because they have several toxic defense mechanisms that damage our digestive systems. Remember, grains are seeds meant to grow, not be digested. That is why they are passed through most animals' digestive systems completely intact. Many of our modern ailments such as asthma, eczema, allergies, migraines, irritable bowl syndrome, leaky gut syndrome and Crohn's disease have been linked to the consumption of both processed and whole grains.

I have personally eliminated all grains from my diet and have had clients do the same with amazing results. Even though corn and quinoa are considered seeds by many in the health and food world, I have also found these to be troublesome to a lot of peoples' digestive systems. I personally consider corn and quinoa to be pseudo-grains, as they cause the same types of health problems that grains do, for most.

The Gluten Question

Gluten is a protein found in numerous grains, cereals, breads, desserts and flours. Gluten cannot be processed correctly in the bodies of people who are allergic to gluten, who are gluten sensitive, and who have celiac disease.

I don't want to go too far into the weeds when talking about gluten, but I think it is an important topic to briefly address. The primary grains that contain gluten are wheat, barley and rye. But here's the catch: Numerous other grains can contain gluten or gluten derivatives, so if you have a sensitivity to gluten it can be fairly difficult to navigate the gluten-free world while continuing to eat other grains. Here's why:

1. Most gluten-free products will contain grains that are considered gluten-free, but actually contain a gluten derivative that can cause the same issues as gluten does for most.

2. Many of these products are corn-based and I have found a large number of people also have problems with corn. Also, ninety-five percent of the corn in the United States is GMO (genetically modified).

Now, that's not to say you can never consume grains again, but just be aware that they can cause great distress to your digestive system and health.

For those looking to really dig into the topic of gluten, I would highly recommend the book *Wheat Belly,* as it has a ton of information on the topic.

7

Does Eating Fat Make You Fat?

Misleading and false information concerning dietary fat has confused many (if not most) of us. Should we eat fat? Any fat? What kind of fat? One thing is certain: In our dietary quest to cut the fat, it's the truth that has most often been removed. We are bombarded with low-fat foods by a food industry that promises to lower our cholesterol and make us thinner and healthier. But, in reality, we are getting fatter and sicker at an alarming rate.

What we can conclude from this charade is that healthy fat is not the culprit. Rather, it is the consumption of vast amounts of high-carbohydrate, low-protein and low-fat food products that is actually making our collective health much worse.

This section will bring misconceptions about fat to an end. Dietary fat is *not* bad and is *not* to be confused with body fat. Rather, fat is an important source of energy and plays many vital roles in all aspects of your health. Read on for the skinny on dietary fat.

COMMON MISCONCEPTIONS ABOUT DIETARY FAT

Almost every day an article comes out expounding the so-called evils of fat, alongside another (contrary) column refuting such claims.

Common myths about dietary fats include:

1. You don't need fat in your diet.

2. To lose weight, it's best to eat low-fat products.

3. Heart disease is mainly caused by excessive saturated fat consumption.

4. Margarine is better than butter for your heart.

5. Excessive dietary fat causes diabetes.

6. Carbohydrates are healthier than natural fats.

7. Meat is bad for you because it contains fat.

8. Dietary fat automatically leads to body fat.

9. Cholesterol-containing foods are bad for you.

Surprised that these are all untrue? Well, the truth about fat runs countercurrent to the vast majority of what mainstream sources say regarding this essential macronutrient.

Herein, we'll examine how fats got a bad rap. We'll also discuss common misunderstandings about the relationship between dietary salt and high blood pressure.

By the end of this section you will understand why the preceding misconceptions are incorrect and how these untruths are detrimental to the average American's health.

Finally, you'll be able to eat your steak, topped with some salt and a bit of butter, as part of a—yes, that's right—healthy and wholesome meal!

Benefits of Fat Consumption

Dietary fat is essential for optimal health.

Fat has several important functions in the human body: as an energy source, in the creation and balance of hormones, in the formation of our cell membranes, in the formation and healthy functioning of our brains and nervous systems, and in the vital transport of fat soluble vitamins (A, D, E and K) within the human body.

Fats are also important for the health of the following organs and systems:

- **Immune system:** Some fats ease and modulate inflammation, helping your immune system and metabolism function properly.

- **Digestion:** Fats slow down digestive processes, providing your body with more time to absorb nutrients. They, therefore, can help maintain and prolong stable energy levels and satiety (a feeling of fullness). Fat-soluble vitamins (A, D, E and K) can only be absorbed by your body when fat is present; these vitamins could otherwise be excreted via your urine and stool.

- **Lungs:** Saturated fat is needed for the proper functioning of lung surfactant (a substance produced by the lungs that helps you breathe normally).

- **Heart:** Certain fats help to maintain a regular heart rhythm. Plus, fat literally keeps your heart ticking. As a primary cardiac fuel source, fat accounts for 60 percent of the heart's fuel supply.

- **Brain:** Fat is essential for proper memory, learning abilities and mood regulation. Sixty percent of the brain is composed of fat. Consuming fat is especially important for pregnant women, since fats are essential to fetal brain development.

- **Cells:** Cell membranes are composed of fatty acids. Fats allow cellular walls to be flexible and healthy, and to retain their normal electrical conductivity.

- **Nerves:** Fats create the material that protects and insulates nerves. This supports the internal communication system of the body by isolating electrical (nerve-based) impulses and speeding their transmission.

- **Eyes:** Fats are essential to eye function and tissue health.

- **Organs:** Fats protect and cushion your internal organs.

Fat: The Hunger-Buster

Removing fats from your diet will increase your hunger levels, since fat is a dense fuel that burns slowly and steadily, providing hours of satiety. This is especially true if your diet is mostly carbohydrate-based, since carbs are digested more quickly than proteins or fats, and may be thought of as emergency fuel that burns fast and is used up just as quickly. Plus, carbs are even faster to digest when eaten without any accompanying fat or protein.

You may have experienced this increase in low-fat-initiated hunger if you have ever fallen victim to the very low-fat or no-fat diets of the past and found yourself ravenous and thinking about food all day.

SATURATED AND UNSATURATED FATS

At its most basic level, a fatty acid is made up of a group of chemical elements such as carbon, oxygen and hydrogen. The group is organized into a chain-like structure, and some of the elements are joined together with links known as chemical bonds. The types of chemical bonds that involve the carbon atoms of a fatty acid are what help determine whether it is a saturated or an unsaturated fat:

- If all of a fatty acid's available carbon bonds are joined to (i.e., *saturated* by) hydrogen atoms, it's called a *saturated* fat.

- If a fatty acid's carbon bonds are *not* occupied by hydrogen atoms, and are instead linked to the other carbon atoms within the fatty acid molecule, the carbon atoms are *unsaturated*. These types of fatty acids are what make up unsaturated fats.

- Both *monounsaturated* fats and *polyunsaturated* fats are types of unsaturated fats. The prefixes *mono* (one) and *poly* (many) refer to the number of carbon-to-carbon chemical bonds in the molecular structure of the fat. Monounsaturated fats have one; polyunsaturated fats have more than one.

It is these differences in chemical structure that give each type of fat its unique characteristics, such as chemical stability (does it go rancid easily?), physical texture (is it liquid or solid at room temperature?), and its ability to withstand heat (is it suited for high-temperature cooking or will it easily burn?).

A special note: Many fats, such as cooking oils, are made up of more than one type of fat. For example, an oil may contain both mono- and polyunsaturated fats. However, for our purposes it is sufficient to describe them in terms of the type of fat that makes up the majority of the cooking oil, and it is this convention that I have followed.

Rancid Fats and Chemical Stability

Chemically speaking, **saturated fats are stable** and tend to not react with other chemicals in their environment, such as the oxygen in the air around us. They tend to last a long time and not "go off," which is why you can keep a tub of cooking lard in the cupboard for months at a time.

In contrast, **unsaturated fats are relatively unstable**, chemically speaking. This means they are more reactive to other chemicals in their environment, such as oxygen in the air (which involves a reaction known as oxidation).

As unsaturated fats break down on a chemical level, they are described as becoming *rancid*. This is why unsaturated cooking oils (such as olive oil) may have a strange or "off" smell after sitting in the cupboard for several months, and become unusable over time.

Texture, Temperature and Cooking with Fats

When at room temperature or refrigerated, **saturated fats are solid or semi-solid** (e.g., butter, lard, coconut oil). Saturated fats are chemically stable at high temperatures and are ideal for use in cooking.

At room temperature, **monounsaturated fats are usually liquid** (e.g., olive oil). Monounsaturated fats may become solid if refrigerated. They are useful for cooking at low to medium temperatures.

At cold temperatures, **polyunsaturated fats are usually liquid** (e.g. flax oil, cod liver oil). At room temperature, polyunsaturated fats are less chemically stable and are therefore usually best stored in the fridge or a cool dark place to prevent rancidity. Polyunsaturated fats are not recommended for use in cooking but may be eaten cold, such as on salads.

THE RIGHT WAY TO USE OILS

Always use unrefined organic oils whenever possible. This means the process of extraction was cold and did not involve the use of high heat and potentially health-sapping hexane gas.

Take advantage of each oil's chemical properties by following these guidelines for use:

Healthy Salad Oil Choices

- Extra virgin olive oil (also okay for cooking up to 325 degrees Fahrenheit)

- Sesame and peanut oils

- Flax oil (in small amounts)

Healthy Cooking Oil Choices

For use **without** heat (stable up to 120 degrees Fahrenheit) e.g., drizzle over vegetables for flavor

- Flax seed oil

- Hemp seed oil

- Cod liver oil

For use with **low** heat (stable up to 212 degrees Fahrenheit)

- Safflower oil

- Sunflower oil

- Pumpkin oil

For use with **medium** heat (stable up to 325 degrees Fahrenheit)

- Sesame oil

- Pistachio oil

- Hazelnut oil

- Olive oil

For use with **high** heat (stable up to 375 degrees Fahrenheit)

- Coconut oil

- Ghee (clarified butter)

- Palm oil

- Avocado oil

- Lard

Sources of Fat

Saturated fats are usually solid or semi-solid at room temperature and are mostly found in animal fats and tropical oils. Examples include butter, coconut or palm kernel oils, and the fat in cheese, full-fat milk and meats.

All meats contain some saturated fat. Pork and beef contain the most. However, chicken, turkey, and fatty fish such as salmon and mackerel also contain saturated fat, albeit much less. Indeed, compared to pork and beef, fatty fish contain minimal amounts. **Monounsaturated fats** are most commonly found in olive oil, as well as the oils of avocados, almonds, cashews, pecans and peanuts. Chicken skin and lard also contain significant amounts.

Polyunsaturated fats tend to remain liquid, even when refrigerated. Examples include sunflower seed oil, canola oil and fish oil, as well as some of the fats contained in eggs and walnuts.

Temperature has an impact on less chemically stable oils, and polyunsaturates in particular. They can easily go rancid and, when heated, oxidize quickly (i.e., lose electrons and become chemically unstable).

For this reason, these fragile fats should only be prepared through traditional cold-press techniques. This occurs when the oil is extracted from the parent seed, grain or nut through compression at the lowest temperature possible. Polyunsaturated cooking oils should only be consumed at room temperature or below, and should never be used for cooking.

Cold-Pressed Oils

Oils that are labeled *cold-pressed* are essentially unrefined oils; no solvents of any kind should be used in their extraction.

Unlike cold-pressed oils, highly processed oils should always be avoided. Why? Many of the cheap, refined oils sold today are derived through the use of chemical solvents. These solvents help to extract more of the oil from the parent source (such as the olive, seed or nut) and increase the oil's stability and shelf life, but these oils are problematic once in the body. In addition, canola oil is almost always derived from genetically modified (GMO) rapeseeds, so as a rule it should always be avoided unless labeled UDSA 100% Organic.

The solution? Always purchase oils that say cold-pressed or virgin on the label, as these are the least refined of all oils. And buy organic whenever you can.

POLYUNSATURATED FATS: OMEGA-3S, OMEGA-6S, AND THEIR IMPACT ON YOUR HEALTH

Two polyunsaturated fats that have received a lot of media attention of late are omega-3 and omega-6 fatty acids. Your body cannot generate these types of fatty acids. Thus, they are termed *essential* fatty acids since they are both required for healthy body functioning and can only be efficiently obtained from the food you eat.

Recently, the benefits of omega-3s such as flax seed oil and fish oil have been heavily promoted by the numerous food and supplement companies that sell them. But before you use any such supplements, let's investigate the facts behind these fats that have incurred so much publicity.

All About Omega-3s

- There are several types of omega-3 fatty acids. These come from both animal and vegetable sources. Two crucial ones—eicosapentaenoic acid (EPA) and docosahexaenoic acid (DHA)—are primarily found in certain types of fish. Plants such as flax contain alpha-linolenic acid (ALA), another kind of omega-3 fatty acid that is partially converted into DHA and EPA in the body. Algae oil often provides only DHA.

- DHA and EPA are found together only in fatty types of fish (such as mackerel, trout and tuna) and algae. Flax seeds and plant sources of omega-3s provide ALA, which is a precursor to EPA and DHA and a source of energy.

- DHA and EPA from fish and fish oil have greater health benefits than plant-based ALA.

Omega-3s confer a number of health benefits. They reduce inflammation throughout the body—in the joints, blood vessels and elsewhere. Omega-3 supplements, such as EPA and DHA, also appear to aid cellular function and to reduce blood viscosity by lowering heart-hostile blood levels of homocysteine (an amino acid that may raise the risk of heart disease).

The Many Benefits of Omega-3 Fatty Acids

- **Dementia and Alzheimer's disease:** Some preliminary research suggests that omega-3s may help protect against Alzheimer's disease and dementia.

- **Asthma:** There is some evidence that fish oil may improve lung function and reduce dependency on medications.

- **Blood pressure and cholesterol:** According to a number of studies, omega-3 fatty acids from fish oil can lower blood pressure. Fish oil can also cut heart disease-predicting triglyceride levels by 20 to 50 percent.

- **Cardiovascular health:** Omega-3 fatty acids appear to lower your overall risk of death from heart disease. Fish oil may reduce arrhythmias (abnormal heart rhythms). People who take omega-3 supplements after a heart attack lower their risk of having a second one. Eating fish once or twice a week also seems to significantly lower the risk of stroke.

- **Osteoporosis:** Studies suggest that foods or supplements containing omega-3s can improve bone density.

- **Rheumatoid arthritis:** Studies have found that omega-3 fatty acids can reduce joint pain and stiffness.

- **Depression:** Cultures that eat foods with high levels of omega-3s seem to have lower levels of depression, some studies show. Fish oil may also help reduce symptoms related to bipolar disorder.

- **Prenatal health:** Studies show when pregnant women take EPA and DHA supplements during pregnancy, they assist in both fetal development and improve the health of their babies. DHA appears to be important for neurological and visual development in infants.

- **Attention deficit hyperactivity disorder (ADHD):** Some studies have found that fish oil can reduce the symptoms of ADHD in school-age children and improve their cognitive function.

- **Other conditions:** Although the quality of supporting evidence varies, some research shows that omega-3s might have a role in treating or reducing the risks associated with many other conditions, such as obesity, painful menstrual cycles, some cancers, lupus, kidney damage due to diabetes, skin conditions and Crohn's disease.

Food and Supplement Sources of Omega-3 Fatty Acids

- Consider eating more free-range poultry, eggs and beef. Free-range animals (animals allowed to graze for food with the sun on their backs in a field or pasture, rather than being enclosed in cages) have much higher levels of omega-3s than typical grain-fed animals (animals that are usually confined and fed cheap grains such as corn and soy as their primary diet).

- Fish high in DHA and EPA omega-3 fatty acids include bluefish, anchovies, mackerel, herring, salmon (wild has much more omega-3s than farmed), sardines, sturgeon, tuna and lake trout. Try to eat these types of fish two to three times a week.

- When possible, try to get omega-3 fatty acids from foods rather than supplements, since natural foods also contain other vital nutrients. With a supplement, you may get adequate omega-3s but miss out on other nutrients and health-boosting cofactors that your body also needs.

- ALA is converted into omega-3 fatty acids in the body. Good food sources of ALA include flax, walnuts, flaxseed oil and olive oil.

All About Omega-6s

Omega-6 fatty acids are also considered to be essential, They are necessary for human health, but the body cannot make them so they must be obtained through dietary sources. Along with omega-3 fatty acids, omega-6 fatty acids play a crucial role in brain function and normal growth and development. They stimulate skin and hair growth, maintain bone health, regulate metabolism and maintain the reproductive system of the body.

A healthy diet contains a balance of omega-3 and omega-6 fatty acids.

The Many Benefits of Omega-6 Fatty Acids

Omega-6 fatty acids can come from food or from supplements. For example, the omega-6 known as gamma-linolenic acid (GLA) is present in evening primrose oil as well as other sources. Below are some health concerns that respond well to these fatty acids:

- **Diabetic neuropathy:** Some studies show that taking gamma-linolenic acid (GLA) for six or more months may reduce symptoms of diabetic neuropathy, including nerve pain. People who have good control over their blood sugar levels may find GLA more effective than those who do not.

- **Breast cancer:** One study found that women with breast cancer who took supplemental GLA had a better response to tamoxifen (a controversial drug used to treat estrogen-sensitive breast cancer) than those who took tamoxifen alone.

- **Mastalgia:** Mastalgia is a mildly discomforting to severely incapacitating form of breast pain. Some evidence suggests that evening primrose oil may reduce breast pain and tenderness in people with cyclic mastalgia. It may also help reduce symptoms to a lesser extent in people with non-cyclic mastalgia. However, it does not seem to be effective in treating breast pain that is severe.

- **High blood pressure (hypertension):** There is some preliminary evidence that GLA may help reduce high blood pressure, either alone or in combination with the omega-3 fatty acids EPA and DHA. In one study, men with borderline hypertension who took six grams of GLA-rich black currant oil experienced a reduction in diastolic blood pressure compared to those who took a placebo.

- **Osteoporosis**: Some studies suggest that people who don't get enough of some essential fatty acids (particularly EPA and GLA) are more likely to suffer bone loss than those with healthy levels of these fatty acids. In a study of women over age 65 with osteoporosis, those who took EPA and GLA supplements had less bone loss over a three-year period than those who took a placebo. Many of these women also experienced an increase in bone density.

- **Premenstrual syndrome (PMS)**: A minority of studies has found that some women report relief of PMS symptoms when taking supplemental GLA. The most improved symptoms have been breast tenderness, feelings of depression and irritability, and swelling and bloating from fluid retention.

- **Multiple sclerosis**: Evening primrose oil has been suggested as a complementary treatment (in addition to standard therapy) for multiple sclerosis (MS), although there is no scientific evidence that backs such claims. MS patients who want to add evening primrose oil to their treatment regimens should first speak with a health care provider.

Food and Supplement Sources of Omega-6 Fatty Acids

Omega-6 fatty acids can be found in a variety of foods and a selection of vegetable oils. Some natural sources of omega-6 fatty acids include walnuts, sesame seeds and oil, cashews, avocados, acai berries and flax seed oil.

Before taking additional omega-6 fatty acids, tell your doctor about any other supplements you take. Omega-6s may interact with other supplements, medications or herbal medicines, including blood thinning drugs, chemotherapy treatment for cancers, and medications such as phenothiazines. Tell your doctor about any supplemental omega-6s you take prior to starting any new pharmaceutical or herbal medication.

How Processed Polyunsaturated Fats Affect Your Health

Unfortunately, the typical American consumes disproportionate amounts of omega-6s if eating commercially produced vegetable oils derived from soy, corn, safflower and canola. Sadly, in many processed foods, healthy animal fats such as butter or lard have been replaced by these omega-6-heavy vegetable oils.

Polyunsaturated fats (such as omega-6s) that originate from vegetable oils have been proven to increase the risk of heart disease and cancer. They also contribute to immune dysfunction, liver damage, digestive disorders, impaired growth and weight gain, amongst other health concerns.

Simple Life Health Point: While polyunsaturated fatty acids are not inherently bad, it is unhealthy to consume them in unreasonable or disproportionate amounts. The sad truth is the typical American diet contains mostly harmful polyunsaturated fats, since highly refined vegetable oils are used as ingredients in the majority of the foods (and especially the processed foods) that Americans consume today.

Why do polyunsaturated fats cause health problems?

It's because of the way they are processed. Polyunsaturated oils become damaged and rancid through both their extraction and during the process of hydrogenation, as described below.

As liquid vegetable oils are chemically and mechanically altered to become semi-solid or solid in consistency, the oils are exposed to high heat, oxygen and moisture levels. Hydrogen is forced into the vegetable oil to change the shape of the molecules, creating a more solid texture. This is how liquid vegetable oils are turned into solid margarine.

Rancid oils, such as these hydrogenated oils, contain free radicals, which are unstable and highly reactive chemicals. Because they are chemically unstable, free radicals tend to cause damage to human tissues and are believed to accelerate the progression of cancer, cardiovascular problems and age-related diseases. Free radicals attack red blood cells and cell membranes in the body, damaging DNA and RNA strands (protein strands that contain your body's genetic blueprint). Research shows that free radicals are directly linked to Alzheimer's disease, autoimmune diseases and skin damage (i.e., wrinkles).

Consuming anything more than small amounts of polyunsaturated oils may contribute to heart disease, cancer, autoimmune diseases, premature aging, learning disabilities and intestinal problems. **We tend to consume enough naturally occurring polyunsaturated oils in a healthy diet through nuts, seeds, certain vegetables and fish oils.** These amounts are not harmful so long as they are from healthy sources and we don't overdo them.

Remember, the consumption of large amounts of polyunsaturated fat is new and unique to the modern industrial diet, due in large part to the widespread prevalence of cheaper liquid vegetable oils, their hydrogenated counterparts, and the plethora of processed foods containing them. Food manufacturers increase their profit line by using these cheaper, damaged oils at the expense of the public's health.

Your current diet may lack foods that contain a healthy balance of omega-3 and omega-6 fatty acids. In a perfect world, we would be able to get adequate and balanced amounts of omega-3s from food sources. However, this is not necessarily possible in today's world. Many vital nutrients are diminished or destroyed in commercially mass-produced foods. So, for some of us, a well-chosen fatty acid supplement is beneficial.

To determine whether or not you need a supplement, consider the symptoms of a deficiency:

- Achy or popping joints (essential fatty acids lubricate the body's joints)

- Dry or brittle hair, fingernails or toenails

- Feeling fatigued and unmotivated

- Irregular bowel movements, constipation, gas or bloating

If you have any of these symptoms, I highly recommend you take an essential fatty acid supplement. Carefully monitor your symptoms thereafter to determine if supplements help to alleviate or reduce your concerns.

I carry a high-quality fish oil supplement under *The Simple Life* label on my website: **www.thesimplelifenow.com**

UNDERSTANDING TRIGLYCERIDES AND HOW THEY AFFECT YOUR HEALTH

If you are like most people, you may have a vague notion that it's a good thing if your doc tells you your triglycerides are low. However, most people don't realize that the lipids known as triglycerides are intimately related to carbohydrate consumption and weight loss. Here are some need-to-know triglyceride facts:

- Most of the fats in our bodies, and in the foods we eat, are made up of triglycerides.

- Triglycerides are a type of lipid (a category of fat-soluble molecules that includes steroids and cholesterol).

- Triglycerides may be kept in your fat cells as a form of long-term energy storage, or travel through the circulatory system to provide energy for essential body functions.

Sources of Triglycerides

Some of the triglycerides in your body come directly from dietary fats. Others have been formed in the liver from excess sugars (mainly fructose) that have not been used for energy (for example, through excess eating and/or lack of exercise). This is how dietary carbohydrates, such as refined sugar and white flour, may contribute to elevated levels of blood-borne triglycerides.

Triglycerides and Weight Loss

The presence of insulin in the bloodstream affects how and when triglycerides are broken down for use and/or stored in fat cells for later use.

Simply, the higher your insulin level, the more triglycerides are released into your bloodstream, greatly increasing your risk of heart disease, obesity, diabetes and hypertension.

TRANS FATS

Trans fatty acids, also known as trans fats, are an artery-clogging, unhealthy type of fat that is formed when vegetable oils are hardened (hydrogenated) into margarine or shortening. Some experts refer to man-made trans fats as "plastic" fats due to their unnatural chemical processing and texture. These plastic fats (hydrogenated trans fats) are very unhealthy and should be avoided at all costs.

Trans fats are found in many industrially produced foods including fried foods (e.g., french fries, fried chicken) and countless commercial baked goods such as doughnuts, cookies, chips, pastries and crackers.

Unfortunately, many food companies use trans fats instead of traditional, healthy, solid baking fats such as butter and coconut oil in order to reduce their production costs, extend the storage life of their products, and mimic the texture of baked goods made with traditional fats.

Hydrogenated trans fats are associated with:

- An increased risk of heart disease

- Impaired immune function

- An inhibition of the body's use of omega-3 fatty acids and the production of long-chain omega-3 fatty acids

- An increased incidence of asthma

- Weight gain

- An increased incidence of cancer

- Infertility

- Clogging of the arteries

- Type 2 diabetes

- A decrease in the optimal functioning of cellular walls

Additionally:

- Dietary trans fats are absorbed into brain cell membranes where they disrupt the cells' ability to communicate with one another.

- Trans fats build up in cell membranes but break down very slowly, and they therefore remain in your body for a long period of time.

- Trans fats are known to increase blood levels of low-density lipoprotein (LDL), the so-called bad cholesterol, while lowering levels of high-density lipoprotein (HDL), also known as good cholesterol.

Simple Life Health Point: Hydrogenated oil-based food products (including many butter substitutes such as margarine) each have a laundry list of negative health effects a mile long, not including any as-of-yet undiscovered concerns. Avoid products containing them at all costs.

Natural versus Unnatural Trans Fats

Unnatural, man-made trans fats are to be avoided like the plastic-fat plague they are. However, trans fats also occur naturally in meat. But take note: This does not mean you need to become a vegetarian. Here's why.

Trans fatty acids are found in very small amounts in the fat of ruminant animals. Ruminant animals are herbivores that primarily eat grass and grass-like vegetation. Examples include cows, as well as antelope, buffalo, deer, goats and sheep. Trans fats make up only between two and five percent of the fat in the meat from these species. Natural trans fats (such as vaccenic acid found in small amounts in dairy and beef fat) have, in fact, been associated with lowering risk factors for diabetes and heart disease.

In contrast, 50 to 60 percent of today's processed and hydrogenated vegetable oils are typically made up of plastic trans fat! This alone should show you that the easiest, most logical way to reduce your trans fat intake is to give up processed carb-based foods made with trans fat-rich hydrogenated oils.

But it's not just about quantity; the quality of trans fats varies as well. The chemical structure of the trans fats found in ruminant animals is far different from the trans fats found in the uber-processed foods that populate grocery shelves. Simply put, the trans fats in ruminant animals are not harmful for you to consume, and your body treats them as a healthy fat.

The bottom line? Pay attention to fat quality (think natural meats, not processed carbs) and the quantity will take care of itself!

Below is a list of some common foods that contain hydrogenated fats (all of which should be avoided!).

- **Candy and cookies:** Look at the labels; some have higher trans or hydrogenated fat content than others. A cookie or a chocolate bar with nuts will likely have more trans fat than gummy bears.

- **Frozen foods:** Most frozen baked products contain trans fat. These include pies, pot pies, waffles, pizzas and even breaded fish sticks. Even if the label says it's a low-fat product, it may still contain unhealthy trans fats.

- **Spreads:** Margarine, non-butter spreads and shortening may all contain large amounts of trans fats.

- **Packaged foods:** Cake, pancake, waffle and other

pre-packaged mixes virtually all have several grams of trans fats per serving.

- **Toppings and dips:** Most non-dairy creamers, flavored coffees, whipped toppings, bean dips, gravy mixes and salad dressings contain large amounts of trans fats, as well as a witch's brew of noxious chemicals.

- **Soups:** Many canned soups and ramen noodles can contain very high levels of trans fats.

- **Fast food:** Bad news here! Fries, chicken and other fast foods are deep-fried in partially hydrogenated oil. Even if the restaurant's kitchen uses liquid oil, fries are sometimes partially fried in trans fat before they're even shipped to individual eateries. Pancakes and grilled sandwiches also contain some trans fats from the margarine that is usually slathered on the grill.

- **Baked goods:** More trans fats are used in commercially baked products than any other foods. Doughnuts contain shortening in the dough and are cooked in trans fats. Frosted cookies and cakes from supermarket bakeries also usually contain plenty of trans fats.

- **Chips and crackers:** Shortening provides a crispy texture to foods. Any foods prepared through frying (such as potato chips and corn chips), or crispy foods like so-called "buttery" crackers, have trans fats. Even reduced-fat brands may still contain trans fats.

- **Breakfast foods:** Virtually all breakfast cereals and energy bars are quick-fix, highly processed products that contain trans fats (even those that claim to be healthy).

This list is especially useful since, shockingly, foods whose labels show "zero" trans fats may still, in actuality, contain the offending lipids. So how are harmful trans fats lawfully concealed from the consumer? As noted on the website of the Federal Drug Administration (FDA) (with my italics):

As of January 1, 2006, food manufacturers must now list trans fat content on nutrition labels. *However, this federal labeling rule allows manufacturers to list "zero" if the product contains less than half of a gram of trans fat per serving.* Therefore, the product could still contain small amounts of shortening or partially hydrogenated vegetable oil while showing zero trans fat. Also, no percentage of daily value (%DV) is listed, as trans fat has no known nutritional value.

Further, the per-serving size listed on nutritional labels is often unrealistically small relative to what most people eat. An actual, real-world serving eaten by the average person might potentially contain many more grams of trans fat than anticipated by an overly conservative label.

Obviously, the best way to avoid trans fats is to completely avoid foods that contain, or are prepared with, highly processed oils—especially hydrogenated and partially hydrogenated oils. Instead, use stable fats for high-heat cooking and baking such as butter, lard and coconut oil, and oils such as olive and flax in their natural (organic) forms for salads and other cold applications.

Trans fats are another negative added to the list of reasons to avoid highly processed foods. Most trans fat-containing foods are high in carbohydrates and sugars to boot. If you avoid processed, sugary, carb-based foods you will almost always be avoiding trans fats as well.

Tackling the Cholesterol Myth

CHOLESTEROL FACTS VERSUS FICTION

For decades now, dietary cholesterol has suffered such scorchingly rotten press that many of us are terrified to even think of eating an egg yolk or a steak. So we reach for those purportedly "heart-healthy" carbs instead. However, this kind of thinking is sadly misguided.

Cholesterol, as it turns out, is naturally produced by the body, is essential for health, and is, as you will discover, quite undeserving of its sinister notoriety. In fact, you would not be able to survive without cholesterol. You would literally die without it!

In this chapter we will discuss:

- Why cholesterol—far from being a dietary evil—is actually a vital and healthful nutrient

- Why the cholesterol in the foods you eat has only a minor effect on measurable levels of blood-borne cholesterol

- Why the terms "good" and "bad" cholesterol are misleading

- How common cholesterol-lowering drugs may do more harm than good

- How pharmaceutical companies profit from misleading you

To begin, we'll cover some technical information on the physiology and chemistry of cholesterol so you can, as always, make your mind up for yourself. We'll conclude by discussing why cholesterol-lowering drugs may not be right for you—or for almost anyone.

Cholesterol chemistry: Cholesterol is made up of a combination of lipids (fats) and sterols, and is most correctly called a lipid alcohol.

Cholesterol: The Vital Nutrient

Since so many of us have been exposed to misleading information about cholesterol, it may be surprising to learn just a few of the ways that it supports your health:

- The cholesterol in cellular membranes makes the cells waterproof, so that there can be a different chemistry on the inside versus the outside of the cell.

- Cholesterol is nature's repair substance.

- Many important hormones are made of cholesterol.

- Cholesterol is vital to the functioning of the brain and nervous system.

- Cholesterol protects us against depression. It plays a role in the utilization of serotonin, the body's "feel-good" chemical.

- Bile salts, needed for the digestion of fats, are made from cholesterol.

- Cholesterol is a precursor of vitamin D, which is formed by the action of ultra-violet (UV-B) light on cholesterol in the skin.

- Cholesterol is a powerful antioxidant that protects us against free radicals and, therefore, against cancer.

- Cholesterol, especially LDL-cholesterol (the so-called bad cholesterol), helps fight infection.

Cholesterol quick fact: Infants need cholesterol for proper brain development. Large amounts of cholesterol are supplied to infants via human milk. In addition, special mammary glands secrete a specific enzyme into human milk to boost the infant's ability to absorb cholesterol.

Does Dietary Cholesterol Cause Unhealthy Cholesterol Levels?

Until recently, dietary cholesterol has gotten a bad rap for ostensibly causing high blood cholesterol levels. This theory is now seriously under attack. Research now tells us that the liver contributes much more cholesterol to the body than do food sources.

In addition, only a small amount of the cholesterol that you eat is actually absorbed into your bloodstream. Your genetic makeup, it turns out, is more of a determinant of your cholesterol levels than your diet.

This being said, there is evidence that, for some people, dietary cholesterol is absolutely essential because their body cannot produce enough for its own use. However, this is the exception rather than the rule.

Dietary versus Blood-Borne (Serum) Cholesterol

To understand these findings, it's important to know the difference between dietary cholesterol and cholesterol of the blood/serum (serum is a liquid component of human blood).

- **Blood/serum cholesterol** is a soft, waxy substance present in all parts of the body, including the brain, nervous system, skin, muscle, liver, intestines and heart. **It is made by the body** and generated from fatty substances in the diet. Cholesterol is made in the liver for later use in normal body functions, including the production of hormones, bile and vitamin D.

- **Dietary cholesterol** is contained **in the foods you eat**. It is mainly found in animal foods such as meat, fish, poultry, eggs, dairy products and shellfish. Organ meats, such as liver, are especially high in cholesterol, while plant-derived foods have none. Once eaten, it serves as a structural component of cell membranes and contributes to other physiological functions.

- About 80 percent of the body's cholesterol is produced in the liver, while the remainder comes from dietary sources.

After a meal, dietary cholesterol is absorbed by the intestine and stored in the liver. The liver is able to regulate cholesterol levels in the bloodstream and can secrete it as needed by the body.

So Is Cholesterol Actually a Good Thing?

If you're surprised to see how helpful and essential cholesterol is for health, then brace yourself. The real story of saturated fat and cholesterol likely runs countercurrent to what you may have been taught. Here's the truth:

- Dietary fats, and especially saturated fats, are not nearly as harmful to our bodies as we may have been told. In fact, we desperately need them for many vital functions in our bodies and for optimal health.

- Since approximately 80 percent of the cholesterol your body uses is made by your liver, dietary sources of cholesterol have little influence in this process. (For people who cannot produce enough cholesterol this is not the case, but again, this is a rare, though dangerous, occurrence.)

- There's nothing to be gained by substituting cholesterol-containing foods such as meat, milk, butter and cheese with high-carbohydrate, low-fat bread items. In fact, much harm can be caused from treading this dangerous dietary path.

To more fully understand why, let's examine a few very misleading labels you have likely heard: so-called good and bad cholesterol categories.

Cholesterol: The Good, the Bad and the Poorly Named

Low-density lipoprotein (LDL cholesterol) is often referred to as the "bad" cholesterol, since elevated levels of a certain variety of LDL cholesterol are associated with an increased risk of coronary heart disease.

High-density lipoprotein (HDL cholesterol) is widely regarded as the "good" form of cholesterol and is often associated with a healthy vascular (blood vessel) system.

But these terms, unfortunately, perpetuate certain misunderstandings about cholesterol itself.

How the Terms "Good" or "Bad" are Misleading

The term *lipoprotein* refers to a biochemical transport assemblage made of proteins and lipids that carries lipids (such as fat and cholesterol) throughout the body in the blood. In short, the transport that delivers cholesterol from the liver to the site of injury is called a low-density lipoprotein (LDL), and the transport that returns the cholesterol to the liver is called a high-density lipoprotein (HDL).

In *Put Your Heart in Your Mouth,* Dr. Natasha Campbell-McBride illuminates the confusion surrounding HDL and LDL cholesterol with a simple analogy:

> *Whenever our liver receives a signal that a wound has been inflicted somewhere in our vascular system, it . . . sends cholesterol to the site of the damage in a shuttle called LDL. Because this cholesterol travels from the liver to the wound in the form of LDL, our "science," in its wisdom, calls LDL a "bad" cholesterol. When the wound heals and the cholesterol is removed, it travels back to the liver in the form of HDL. Because this cholesterol travels away from the artery back to the liver, our misguided "science" called it "good" cholesterol. This is like calling an ambulance traveling from the base to the patient a "bad" ambulance, and the one traveling from the patient back to the base a "good" ambulance.*

WHAT DO CHOLESTEROL LEVELS REALLY MEASURE?

Cholesterol is a major antioxidant that can protect and repair damaged blood vessels. **As you age, you are subject to more free radical activity throughout the body and, in response, the body produces more cholesterol to help contain and control the damage.** It is probably for this reason that serum cholesterol levels tend to naturally rise with age, and also why low cholesterol in an older person is a possible warning signal of a degenerative disease such as cancer.

Since the body uses cholesterol to repair and protect itself from sources of inflammation, a person who improves his or her health through positive lifestyle or dietary changes will tend to have lower serum cholesterol levels because the body no longer needs the extra circulating cholesterol, and because the desired repairs have successfully healed.

Mother's Milk High in Cholesterol and Fat, Vital for Health and Growth

A mother's milk provides a higher proportion of cholesterol than almost any other food. Over half its calories come from fat—much of it saturated fat. Both cholesterol and saturated fat are essential for growth in babies and children, especially for the rapid development of the brain.

Commercial milk-replacement formulas are low in saturated fats, and soy formulas are devoid of cholesterol (plant sterols are often called "plant cholesterol," but they act completely differently from the cholesterol in mother's milk). Sadly, a recent study linked low-fat diets with failure to thrive in children.

How are Cholesterol Levels Measured?

When doctors talk about your "cholesterol levels," they are referring to the amount of blood cholesterol circulating in your body. These levels may be measured as part of medical tests such as a *lipid profile*: a blood analysis that measures your HDL (so-called good cholesterol), LDL (so-called bad cholesterol), triglycerides and total cholesterol. Remember, both cholesterol and triglycerides are categorized as lipids (a broad category of molecules that also includes fats).

Total cholesterol is the sum of

- LDL (low-density) cholesterol

- HDL (high-density) cholesterol

- VLDL (very low-density, oxidized and therefore potentially harmful) cholesterol

- IDL (intermediate-density) cholesterol

THE CHOLESTEROL HYPOTHESIS

Here's where it gets really interesting. The *cholesterol hypothesis* states that if you have high serum cholesterol, you are more likely to acquire coronary heart disease. However, there is very little evidence to support this theory. Numerous studies have shown that people with mid to high levels of cholesterol are just slightly more likely to have coronary heart disease, or a heart attack, as compared to their low-cholesterol measuring counterparts. Indeed, there are too many other health risk factors (smoking, poor exercise habits, high stress, poor diet and so on) that make it difficult to substantiate a direct connection between high cholesterol markers and heart disease.

A mere thirty years ago, a total serum cholesterol level of 300 mg/dl (measured in milligrams of cholesterol per deciliter of blood) was considered normal. These longstanding, normative cholesterol levels are associated with increased longevity, and yet have become pathologically high by today's standards.

Today the normal range has since been lowered to between 200 and 240 mg/dl, despite the fact that in older women it is completely normal and healthy for blood/serum cholesterol levels to be greater than 240 mg/dl. This arbitrary change, based on pharmaceutical sales strategies, automatically resulted in millions of people being suddenly turned into patients in need of "treatment."

Since 1984, in the United States and other parts of the Western world, normal cholesterol levels have been treated as if they were an indication of a disease in progress or a potential for disease in the future. The truth, as previously noted, is that the criteria for "normal" cholesterol levels have increased over the years because of new research findings—research that does not stand up to the bright light of critical analysis.

These skewed figures mean that many doctors have been treating their patients with truly normal cholesterol levels as if they had signs of disease. Unfortunately, many of those who fall victim to this situation are being prescribed medications with numerous dangerous side effects. If such medications were only inexpensive and not life threatening, their use could undoubtedly be shrugged off as a (relatively) harmless snake oil pharmaceutical scam.

However, these are, in fact, thoroughly dangerous drugs with both physical and emotional consequences. All of this has led to a virtual epidemic of cholesterol medicine prescriptions, and the rise of potentially dangerous side effects.

CHOLESTEROL AND MEDICATION: STATINS

Cholesterol is definitely a hot-button health issue in today's society. Moreover, cholesterol-lowering drugs are the best-selling medicines in history, which makes statins big business, with an estimated $19.2 billion of them sold in 2017.

Statins are used by more than 15 million Americans and an additional 12 million other patients worldwide. With the support of drug companies, doctors have also promoted and prescribed cholesterol-treating statins to children as young as eight years old. This is of particular concern when you know the dire consequences that such medication can have, especially on the development of the child's brain. Remember, cholesterol is essential for a child's proper brain development.

Some statin users report memory loss, mood swings, behavioral changes and difficulty concentrating. Other reported side effects have been described as Alzheimer's disease-like cognitive defects, including day-long bouts of amnesia. Statins can lead to serious and potentially untreatable diseases such as liver cancer and muscle disorders, including those involving the heart muscle. Many patients are emotionally and mentally affected by these medications as well.

The Dangers of Statins

A paper published in the *American Journal of Cardiovascular Drugs* (2008) cites nearly 900 studies showing the adverse effects of statins. Some of the findings are outlined below.

The main problem with statins is they do not tend to cause immediate side effects. These drugs are capable of lowering cholesterol levels by as much as 50 points or more. So, on the surface, the patient sees immediate positive results. However, health problems that appear in the future are frequently not correctly identified as a side effect of the drug, but are erroneously deemed new and separate health problems.

Statin use is not benign. Some of the possible side effects of taking statins in strong doses, or for a lengthy period of time, include:

- Cognitive impairment

- Neuropathy (nerve damage)

- Anemia

- Acidosis (increased acidity of the blood and body tissues)

- Frequent fevers

- Cataracts

- Sexual dysfunction

Other serious and potentially life-threatening side effects include, but are not limited to:

- An increased risk of cancer

- Immune system suppression

- Serious degeneration of muscular tissues, including the heart (i.e., rhabdomyolysis)

- Pancreatic dysfunction

- Hepatic dysfunction (due to the potential increase in liver enzymes, patients taking statins must be monitored for normal liver function)

Who Benefits: You or the Pharmaceutical Companies?

In short, drug companies want you to buy cholesterol-lowering drugs (such as statins) so that you think you are lowering your cholesterol, or are even preventing a future heart attack. As long as you follow this suggestion, drug companies will continue to sell you something you don't really need.

Many individuals who have taken statins have told me that their doctors prescribed these medications as the primary method to treat their supposed high cholesterol, but never prescribed a healthy diet or exercise as an alternate option before issuing medication. What's worse? Certainly no one investigated the underlying reasons why they may have exhibited high cholesterol readings (i.e., an inflammatory condition that did, in fact, warrant attention).

A Real Story of Statin Use From a Client

I started having annual physicals about five years ago in an effort to better monitor my overall health. At age 37, I was found to have an average cholesterol level (170 to 200), but a high level of low-density lipids (LDL, the so-called "bad" kind of cholesterol). Despite my best efforts to improve an already decent diet, I could not change my LDL level or my "good" cholesterol (HDL), so my doctor prescribed a low dose (5 mg) of the statin medication Crestor.

Statins can adversely affect liver function, but my doctor had confirmed that Crestor was not affecting my liver. This dosage knocked down my LDL and boosted my HDL. All was well. But I was now taking this little pill every day, and perhaps for the rest of my life. When asked about side effects, my doctor stated that, apart from the potential liver function issue, there were no known side effects. That, of course, could change in the future, as it has with other medications.

A few years later, after getting some chest pains and going through a CT scan of my heart, I was found to have zero arterial build-up. Good news. The cardiologist that ordered the CT scan also did a risk assessment for me with the use of a Framingham cardiac risk score. He was informed of my statin use and was curious as to whether I really needed it.

In the end, the cardiologist found that, despite a little bit of health history on my mother's side, the use of Crestor was not going to greatly decrease my risk of a cardiac issue in the future. Based on its marginal benefit to my overall health, and given all the other factors at play, I decided to stop taking Crestor.

From this experience I learned that taking a medication long-term, despite its perceived benefit, should be a decision that's considered carefully. My primary doctor was focused on knocking down my cholesterol, but it ended there. As I discovered in my case, it turned out that the benefit did not outweigh the risk.

John H.

A Final Thought

The incestuous relationship between the medical community and drug companies is clear and apparent. Keep in mind that drug companies are businesses whose bottom line is to make a profit and keep shareholders happy with ever-increasing sales. Good health does not increase their revenues, but poor health does… and you are the one ultimately paying the real price!

None of this is to say you should simply stop taking your cholesterol-lowering medications. Rather, try incorporating exercise into your lifestyle and improving your diet first.

The Importance of Protein in Maintaining a Healthy Weight

The word *protein* comes from the Greek word *proteios,* which means *of the first importance.* Fittingly, protein is involved in every biological process in the human body.

In our carb-heavy world, it's important to remember that protein is an essential part of our diets. Our bodies use it to repair muscle, grow tissue, regulate hormones, assist with metabolic control, defend against illness and assist in healing wounds. Every cell in the body is partly comprised of protein and is constantly exposed to wear and tear. Regular protein consumption is vital to help repair and replace these cells.

Protein makes up your ligaments, tendons, muscles, hair, nails, skin, teeth, tissue, organs and bones. Of all the non-water mass in your body, 75 percent is made up of protein.

Enzymes—the managers of all of our biochemical processes—are specialized proteins, as are illness-fighting antibodies. Insulin is a protein and, as we have discussed in depth, the management of insulin is unquestionably important in the quest for a slimmer, healthier body.

Protein, in short, is necessary for life.

Probably the best (albeit morbid) example of the importance of dietary protein is the true story of those aboard an airplane that crashed into the Andes Mountains in 1972 (made famous by the 1993 movie *Alive*). To live, the crash survivors had to consume the flesh of those who had died in the plane wreck. They were able to survive solely on human flesh for 72 days. However, without this valuable source of protein and fat, they would surely have perished within weeks. Here's why.

PROTEIN IN THE LIVES OF PRIMITIVE HUMANS

Our ancestors lived as hunter-gatherers for approximately 84,000 generations and some 2.4 million years, the *American Journal of Medicine* recently noted. But here is substantial food for thought: Our primitive counterparts survived mostly on a diet of meat and fat, supplemented by vegetables, fruits, seeds and nuts. Studies of ancient remains show that these primitive peoples typically had excellent bone structure, heavy musculature and flawless teeth. Many had incredibly thick skulls and strong teeth in relation to modern-day humans.

Most ancient cultures ate a varied diet which included roots, berries, large and small game, insects, scavenged meat and, in some instances, other humans. Without the benefit of modern farming and agriculture, they did not have the ability to consume only one type of food, such as corn, for the entirety of a year. Instead, natural food availability dictated the specific content of their diets. They ate what was naturally abundant and in-season.

For many of these cultures, this meant a truly seasonal menu, since fruits and vegetables do not typically flourish year-round except in tropical regions. Foods from animal sources, such as meat, were a necessity for many, especially those living in colder climates. Clearly, meat, eggs and, to a lesser extent, dairy products were important parts of human life well before the first diet book was ever written.

This seasonal cycle created a balanced diet. Without easy access to calorie-dense convenience foods, our early ancestors ate because of true hunger. This was survival at its most basic: eating to live, not living to eat. Perhaps this is a principle we would do well to understand again.

The good news is that meat from traditionally raised animals is good for you, and you don't have to feel guilty about eating it. Plus, you don't have to go find it, kill it or even butcher it like pre-historic humans did if you choose not to. However, only a handful of companies produce the majority of the commercial, factory-farmed meat in the U.S. While the workings of mass meat production are beyond the scope of this writing, watch out for future projects from *The Simple Life* that will reveal the importance of natural meats and other organic foods.

Simply, you should purchase humanely, organically raised meat whenever possible and economically feasible. I personally only purchase organic meat from local farmers when possible, but I know this is not always feasible for everyone. Just do the best you can. But I urge you to consider going organic. Trust me, your health will greatly improve from this choice.

THE BUILDING BLOCKS OF PROTEIN: AMINO ACIDS IN THE HUMAN BODY

Like carbohydrates and fats, proteins are made up of carbon and hydrogen molecules arranged in specific ways. An amino acid is the smallest unit (or building block) of a protein. When amino acids are joined together, they form peptides (also known as peptide chains). These peptide chains form the primary structure of protein. Unlike other macronutrients, such as fat and carbohydrates, protein also contains nitrogen within its amino acid groups.

In humans, amino acids are involved in energy production; hormone synthesis, activation and release; the production of ammonia and urea (a component of urine); and the regulation of proteins. They also have health-boosting antioxidant properties.

Even though numerous amino acids are found in nature, only 20 different amino acids are found in the human body. **All proteins in your body are made up of a combination of these 20 amino acids, which are categorized as either *essential* or *non-essential*.** These 20 amino acids are commonly found in animal-based sources of dietary protein.

The Eight (or Nine) Essential Amino Acids

Of all of the 20 amino acids that are found in the human body, only nine are considered to be *essential*. This means they are required for physiological functions, yet can only be obtained from the food you consume.

However, many biology and biochemistry texts list only eight essential amino acids. This is because the ninth, histidine, has only recently been labeled as semi-essential. Research now shows that histidine is essential only for some people—specifically, for infants and competitive athletes with rigorous training schedules—which explains its new, in-between classification.

For continuity in our discussion, and because this program deals with the health of average adults (as opposed to infants or high-level athletes), I will defer to the traditional reference of eight essential amino acids. However, be aware that if you work out at a particularly intense level, you will also need to consider histidine in your nutritional plans.

The Eleven Non-Essential Amino Acids

The remaining 11 amino acids can be generated within the human body, if the essential amino acids are already present in the proper amounts. Two of these—cysteine and tyrosine—are sometimes considered to be semi-essential (more on this follows).

If someone is deficient in any of the essential amino acids, his or her body will be unable to produce the other proteins it needs, even when overall protein consumption is high. This is why it is essential for weight-loss and health enthusiasts to consume protein, and especially animal proteins when possible.

Cysteine and Tyrosine: A Special Case of Semi-Essentials

Cysteine and *tyrosine* are two amino acids that, while usually classified as non-essential amino acids, are sometimes considered semi-essential. This is because if you eat sufficient amounts of cysteine and tyrosine (from meat, milk, fish, poultry and legumes, for example), the body can use them in place of two other essential amino acids (methionine and phenylalanine, respectively).

COMPLETE AND INCOMPLETE PROTEINS

Consuming protein (and, therefore, amino acids) every day is essential to your overall health and ability to function. This is because your body is able to maintain relatively stable levels of carbohydrates and fats. But it cannot maintain a consistent amino acid supply pool without a regular dietary supply.

The relative quantity of any one essential amino acid, as compared to all the others, forms a metaphorical bottleneck for your overall nutritional status. Therefore, you must have both an adequate intake of, and relative balance among, the amino acids you eat.

Simple Life Health Point: The most limited essential amino acid you consume affects how well your body uptakes and uses the remaining amino acids. Thus, you should eat some of all eight essential amino acids each day, most easily found in complete proteins from animal sources.

Nutritionally speaking, food sources of protein are generally referred to as either *complete* or *incomplete*:

- A **complete protein** contains all eight essential amino acids.

- An **incomplete protein** only contains some of the eight essential amino acids.

Almost all complete proteins come from animals. Examples include meat, fish, eggs and dairy products. In contrast, vegetables, beans and other plant products contain incomplete proteins, since they do not have all eight essential amino acids.

So what happens when you don't eat complete proteins? To answer this properly, you must understand that **your body cannot store *essential* amino acids for later use**. So, if you don't eat sufficient levels of essential amino acids, your body turns inward and cannibalizes protein from the only source it can: your own muscles. You become weaker as a consequence.

Simple Life Health Point: Incomplete proteins contain only some of the eight essential amino acids. If you don't get essential amino acids from complete protein sources (which have all of the essential amino acids), your body may actually lose muscle instead of building it.

Just one day of insufficient essential amino acid consumption can wreak havoc on your muscles and, as a consequence, your fitness! It is imperative for the right kinds and amounts of protein to be included in your diet.

To ensure this happens, I typically start my day with all eight essential amino acids right out of the gate. I eat a breakfast consisting primarily of complete proteins such as eggs or meat, and include vegetables for fiber and other nutrients. That way I know that, no matter what my day throws at me, I have already eaten all the essential amino acids and have prevented my muscles from being sacrificed to supply these critical nutrients.

Complete Proteins and Vegetarianism

I know some current or former vegetarians will object to some of the aforementioned statements and claim that complete proteins can also be found in plant sources. This is true to an extent; **you can combine two or more vegetarian sources of incomplete proteins** to create a complete set of amino acids within a meal.

Known as forming *complementary proteins*, this technique might include pairing beans with brown rice, corn, wheat or nuts. So, in theory, a meat-free diet can still deliver plenty of dietary protein. However, here's the problem: All vegetarian protein sources also contain a lot of carbohydrates relative to their complete protein content.

So guess what happens? As a vegetarian who faithfully combines complementary plant protein sources, you would still have insulin spikes and an increased propensity to gain body fat. You would also likely be hungry all the time, due to a lack of healthy fats and animal protein that would otherwise reliably provide satiety and contentment. That's why I recommend eating animal products as a healthy way to stay lean and fit.

I do want to make one thing clear: If you're leaning more toward a vegetarian or vegan diet, most of the principles I outline in this book can still be applied. Obviously, you'll have to eliminate or alter the primary protein sources (animal meat or products from animals), but it can still be done.

QUALITY AND QUANTITY OF PROTEIN INTAKE: PRACTICAL APPLICATIONS

The quality of the protein you eat is very important. As in the case of carbohydrates, if you consume highly processed proteins you could develop health problems from the chemical additives contained therein, as well as from the processed (damaged) amino acids themselves.

Also, one protein I try to avoid as much as possible is soy. The main reason I'm opposed to soy is that most soy crops today are genetically modified (GMO). GMO soy foods become toxic in the body and mimic its hormones. This is detrimental to health since natural hormone regulation is a major part of your overall well-being. Plus, you are already inundated with soy products. Soy is added to many seemingly non-soy related, everyday foods, such as salad dressing. It is even used as feed for animals that we will later eat. There are so many other more healthy proteins available that there is no reason to eat a potentially harmful one that also packs its own problems with digestibility and allergies.

To help you assess the quality of your protein intake, a list of healthy and unhealthy protein sources follows below. This will help you determine whether the addition or elimination of certain proteins would be appropriate for your diet. Remember that meat typically contains more fat than vegetarian protein sources, but that this protein-fat combo is the best, most natural way to eat to allow vital nutrients to be absorbed.

Healthy Protein Sources

- Meat (non-processed)

- Organ meats (from wild or pastured animals)

- Fish (wild-caught)

- Whole milk, cheese, yogurt and cottage cheese

- Almond butter

- Nuts

- Eggs

Unhealthy Protein Sources

- Fish (farmed)

- Processed meat (lunch meat, sausage, chicken nuggets, hotdogs, etc.)

- Sugar-filled protein bars

- Soy products

- Fried meat (although bacon is okay on occasion)

HOW PROTEIN-BASED DIETS HELP KEEP YOU THIN

Like many people, you may find it difficult to overeat or binge on foods that contain lots of protein and fat. However, with carbohydrates we don't seem to have that same physiological reaction. When we consume large amounts of carbohydrates, we seem to be able to eat, eat and eat. Hunger overtakes us, and we become ravenous for more. Researchers have studied the metabolic component of hunger, and they made two important observations.

This is one of the main reasons *The Simple Life Healthy Lifestyle Plan* doesn't focus on calories alone. Understanding how calories work has its place (I'll discuss this in detail in the next chapter). However, the caloric volume of your food intake is just one of many factors to consider when it comes to health and weight control.

PROTEIN SUPPLEMENTS

In a perfect world, you'd eat only organic, natural whole food sources of protein without any kinds of powders. But in the real world, the demands of family and work often mean we're eating less-than-ideal meals. A high-quality protein powder, occasionally used, can be an excellent way of closing the gap between the ideal and the real.

At one extreme, we live in a fast-food world dominated by empty carbs. At the other extreme, bodybuilding lore and so-called fitness magazines extol the purported fat-blasting virtues of the powdered protein supplement du jour. How can you wade through the hype and make the right choices for you?

To start, you need an understanding of what goes into protein supplements. These can have a useful place in your fitness routine, but only when you choose well and use them properly. In this spirit, we'll begin by zooming in on the chemical structure of protein supplements so you can wade through the hype and help cut the fat.

Dietary supplements are vitamins, minerals, herbs and other substances meant to boost your nutritional intake. They may take the form of pills, capsules, powders or liquids. Protein powders are one example.

In our modern, often overly-scheduled world, when a healthy meal option is not available, a high-quality protein powder is a great option. Unfortunately, many people purchase the cheapest options available to supplement their organic foods diets. That's like using rusty bent nails to hold together a deck made of the finest woods. It won't work.

You must choose dietary supplements with tremendous care. Many are designed to do only one thing: to make you believe you need them in order to be healthy. However, the only thing they inarguably do is make your wallet lighter.

There's another reason to be careful when purchasing protein powders: Natural carbohydrates and fats can be devitalized through commercial processing and refining, and the same is true of proteins. Isolated protein powders made from soy, whey, casein and egg whites are frequently created via high-temperature processing methods.

This heat alters the natural structure of the proteins until they become virtually unusable by—and even harmful to—the body (this chemical process is called a *denaturing* of the proteins).

As you can see, there are numerous cheaply produced protein drinks and powders that may, in fact, introduce illness and toxic contaminants into our lives. I emphasize this point since the overuse of inferior protein powders is especially prevalent amongst busy folks who want to get fit.

The best way to get a high-quality protein powder is to make sure it is *cold-processed* (this will not denature the protein like heat-processed versions) and *micro-filtered*. Also, when it comes to whey protein, grass-fed is the best choice. For other protein powder options, such as egg- and plant-based versions, try to buy organic.

The supplement industry is booming in the United States, to the tune of an estimated 36 billion dollars spent in 2017 alone. This translates to approximately $100 dollars spent on supplements per person each year.

Not only is the supplement industry in the U.S. big business, but it is also very loosely regulated. Most people believe when they purchase a supplement that it has been highly scrutinized and deemed safe by some federal agency such as the U.S. Food and Drug Administration (FDA) or U.S. Department of Agriculture (USDA). However, nothing could be further from the truth.

This is why I—a former FDA investigator—am meticulously careful about which supplements I use myself! The supplement industry is seen as the Wild West of nutrition by many experts, including myself, because of the scanty oversight that it receives. It's truly buyer beware! We'll discuss this at-length in a subsequent section of this book, but here's what you need to know for now.

THE RIGHT WAY TO EAT PROTEIN

Keep quality and quantity in mind as we discuss the details of how to best include protein in your diet.

In theory, your body can only process and digest up to 30 to 40 grams of protein per meal—or so says a commonly promoted guideline. I have researched this claim and have been unable to find any information to back it up. So why would this assertion exist?

My belief is that when you consume 30 to 40 grams of protein you will feel full. Indeed, you basically have to force yourself to eat more protein than this, a situation that limits most people to less than 40 grams of protein per meal. Plus, most protein is accompanied with fat, which is also nutrient- and calorie-dense, and which helps you feel full and satisfied with your meal.

Forcing oneself to eat more protein, despite feeling full, is a common technique used by bodybuilders striving to gain muscle mass. However, I do not recommend you use this technique. Trust me, in my younger years I did this in order to try to gain muscle like my bodybuilding heroes. Suffice to say, the pain, bloating and frequent trips to the bathroom that this method ushered into my life were unhealthy and, more importantly, unnecessary!

So how much meat and protein should you eat? Well, the days of eating 32-ounce steaks are gone, which is two pounds of meat! My stomach hurts just thinking about that. To start, the portions of meat that you eat should be smaller than what you see in restaurants and in food ads. To keep things simple, try to make a portion of meat match the approximate size of your fist. This portion will be around four to six ounces of meat per meal.

Try also to have some type of complete protein with each of your three main meals, such as eggs, fish, chicken or beef. Include some other proteins such as yogurt, cheese or nuts in your snacks and smaller meals throughout the day.

As I hinted at the beginning of this section, here is my opinion through years of working with clients on how much protein you should consume: I have found that, for most people, around .5 to .75 grams per pound of body weight is more than adequate. For competitive athletes, .75 to 1 gram of protein per pound of body weight is more reasonable, though I've worked with college-level football offensive linemen weighing in the 300-lbs range, and getting them to consume 300 grams of protein per day is pretty much impossible.

Note that the more muscular or active you are, the more protein you will need in order to maintain your current level of strength. You will have to experiment to determine your protein levels since they should be based on your muscle mass and weight, and whether or not you are trying to maintain or increase your muscle mass.

The amount of meat you should eat also depends on your genetic makeup and on hormonal factors. Some people need a lot of dietary protein. However, others are not able to produce adequate levels of hydrochloric acid in their stomachs to break down and digest large amounts of meat. Everyone's different. In my experience, people who eat the correct diet of healthy organic foods often begin to produce enough acid to digest animal meat without any issues.

Moreover, individual requirements for essential amino acids vary greatly. For example, people with darker skin may need more tryptophan, which is found in eggs and dairy products, since this essential amino acid is used in the production of melanin (a substance that gives skin and hair its color). Conversely, some people have high dietary requirements for carnitine (a non-essential amino acid found in lamb and beef) since they have difficulty manufacturing enough on their own for healthy cardiac function.

PROTEIN AND EXERCISE

Your body is made up of approximately 20 percent protein, of which 15 to 20 percent may be used for energy. In athletes, this figure can be as high as 50 percent. In other words, carbohydrates are certainly not the sole source of energy for your body, despite what you may have been taught.

You constantly lose amino acids via exercise, muscular contractions and movement, all of which stimulate the use of protein stores (known as *protein metabolism*). This is why athletes regularly eat large quantities of complete proteins to maintain easy-to-access supplies of amino acids for muscle repair, growth and energy.

In contrast, if your amino acid intake falls below the amount required for your activity level, your body will cannibalize your internal sources of protein, such as enzymes and structural proteins. This commonly occurs in conjunction with overtraining, leading to fatigue and muscle loss.

For example, you may have seen someone in the gym who trains for hours yet never seems to get stronger. He or she is also likely to have less muscular tone than expected for such a level of exercise. Odds are, he or she is overtraining and does not consume enough protein to repair, maintain or build more muscle tissue.

Simple Life Health Point: The post-workout period is the most important opportunity to eat for muscle gains. Working out with weights breaks down your muscle tissue, and supplying protein helps promote growth and rebuilding. In this case, high-quality protein shakes are a practical on-the-go way to get the protein you need.

Is There Such a Thing as Too Much Protein?

We know some protein is good for us, but is there such a thing as too much? There are two common questions in this vein that I'd like to address: whether it is even possible to overeat protein, and whether eating large amounts of protein can cause health problems. We'll tackle these questions in order below.

1. Is it possible to eat protein to excess?

The simple answer to this question is no. If you eat a diet with healthy fats and proteins (which are almost always eaten together, since healthy protein sources usually also contain fats), it is very difficult to eat too much protein.

Here's why: Healthy proteins and fats are satiating (they make you feel full). In contrast, refined carbohydrates make you feel hungry soon after you eat them.

You can see this for yourself quite easily in a simple experiment: Spend one day trying to eat as much healthy protein (with the accompanying fat) as you possibly can, with no carbohydrates except for high-fiber vegetables that are low on the glycemic index (i.e., are absorbed slowly into the bloodstream). Then, for one full day eat as many empty, highly processed carbohydrates as you can (with no healthy protein or fat) and notice the difference in how you feel.

Skeptics who try this short experiment are always amazed at the results. In my experience, they report that it was impossible for them to overeat healthy proteins and fats because they felt full very quickly and stayed full for a long time. But when eating highly processed carbohydrates, they ate and ate all day long without ever feeling satisfied.

When you eat proteins and fats you don't get the insulin spikes that often accompany foods rich in refined carbohydrates. Feeling stuffed and then quickly ravenous again is an unhealthy cycle associated with overeating carbs; this cycle is eliminated when proper amounts of protein and fat are regularly included in your daily diet and you then feel satiated with reasonable portions of food.

There are some people, however, for whom this is not true. Some people have a dysfunction of a portion of the brain called the hypothalamus. The hypothalamus is a small endocrine (hormone-regulating) organ at the base of the brain that plays a crucial role in many physiological functions, including hunger and satiety. For these people, the above does not apply. However, this condition is incredibly rare.

2. Does eating too much protein put pressure on the kidneys and cause health problems?

The simple answer, again, is no. However, I have heard this fallacy for decades, especially from people who love to eat carbohydrates! I have researched this issue extensively and have not been able to find any credible research demonstrating that eating excessive protein causes kidney or health problems. However, I have found numerous studies disproving this idea.

Concerns as to whether consuming high levels of protein is healthy for humans are usually based on the fact that individuals with renal (kidney) disease and renal failure experienced a worsening of kidney function when eating a high-protein diet. However, recent research has shown that individuals with healthy kidneys who eat high levels of protein experience no renal stress and tolerate the increased protein well. In addition, the theories that calcium loss and kidney stones are the result of a high-protein diet have been unsubstantiated.

People with preexisting kidney problems may have to lower their levels of protein intake. However, our discussion is limited to the diets of healthy individuals, and in such instances the latter recommendations do not apply.

A well-known study performed by the University of Connecticut's Department of Nutritional Sciences and published in

Nutrition and Metabolism (2005) concluded the following (with my notes in square brackets):

Recent trends in weight-loss diets have led to a substantial increase in protein intake by individuals. As a result, the safety of habitually consuming dietary protein in excess of recommended intakes has been questioned. In particular, there is concern that high protein intake may promote renal damage by chronically increasing glomerular pressure and hyperfiltration [i.e., by increasing the workload of the kidneys].

There is, however, a serious question as to whether there is significant evidence to support this [hypothetically damaging] relationship in healthy individuals. In fact, some studies suggest that hyperfiltration, the purported mechanism for renal damage, is a normal adaptive mechanism that occurs in response to several physiological conditions.

We researched the available evidence that increased dietary protein intake is a health concern in terms of the potential to initiate or promote renal disease. While protein restriction may be appropriate for treatment of existing kidney disease, we find no significant evidence for a detrimental effect of high protein intakes on kidney function in healthy persons after centuries of a high-protein Western diet.

WHAT ABOUT DAIRY AS A HEALTHY PROTEIN SOURCE?

We frequently think of milk and other dairy products as rich sources of calcium. However, dairy products are also excellent sources of protein. They can add variety for those who prefer not to rely on meat as their sole source of protein. Many animals can, and do, produce milk fit for human consumption. However, cow's milk is one of the healthiest varieties for both children and adults.

The practice of drinking cow's milk is thought to date back from 6,000 to 8,000 B.C. Milk and other dairy products were so highly valued in ancient Egypt that only the very wealthy could afford to consume them. In the fifth century A.D., cow's and sheep's milk became especially prized in Europe. However, it wasn't until the fourteenth century that the demand for cow's milk began to outpace that of sheep's milk. Dairy cows were later brought from Europe to America in the early seventeenth century.

The Benefits of Natural Dairy Foods

Cow's milk provides around eight grams of protein in a one-cup serving and is a good source of low-cost, high-quality protein. This represents 16.3 percent of the recommended daily amount of protein for a healthy adult (remember, this will vary depending on your weight and physical activity).

Milk is also a good source of iodine, calcium, vitamin D, riboflavin, phosphorus, vitamin B_{12}, vitamin K, potassium and vitamin A.

Healthy products made from milk include:

- Cream

- Cream cheese

- Sour cream

- Cheese

- Butter

- Yogurt

- Cottage cheese

Milk supports the health of your bones, skin and immune system, and helps prevent health concerns such as hypertension, dental decay, dehydration, respiratory problems, obesity, osteoporosis, and even some forms of cancer. Unprocessed milk helps prevent anemia (iron deficiency) and osteoporosis (a disease in which the bones become weak and are more likely to break). It is considered the best and most practical source of calcium for all age groups.

Why Some People Can't Consume Dairy

While dairy products are healthy and long-enjoyed staples of the human diet, not everyone can eat them. What follows are some of the reasons why.

Lactose Intolerance

Some people have a low tolerance to pasteurized milk because they lack intestinal lactase, the enzyme that digests lactose (the sugar naturally found in milk). All baby mammals produce lactase, but production of the enzyme declines and may even disappear after weaning. In humans, a mutation or recessive gene allows the production of lactase beyond infancy in some individuals. It is estimated that only 30 to 40 percent of the world's population produces lactase in adulthood.

The overuse of antibiotics also contributes to lactose intolerance. However, some who are considered lactose-intolerant can consume *raw* milk products without problems, as un-pasteurized milk contains the enzyme lactase, and cultured raw milk products (such as yogurt) have consumed the lactose in the fermentation process.

Casein Intolerance

Casein is a protein commonly found in cow's milk, and products derived from it, that can cause some people health problems. Casein is also found in other mammals' milk, but we'll focus on cow's milk for simplicity. A casein intolerance or allergy is different from lactose intolerance, in that lactose intolerance is caused by a partial or complete lack of the digestive enzyme lactase in your body, whereas a casein intolerance or allergy is caused by your body's inability to recognize casein, which causes an immunological response.

An intolerance or allergy to casein can cause the following symptoms:

- Hives

- Rashes

- Wheezing

- Severe pain

- Food malabsorption

- Vomiting

- Breathing problems

- Swelling of the lips, mouth, tongue, face or throat

- Nasal congestion, sneezing, runny nose, and itchy eyes

In my experience, the best way to tell if you have a casein intolerance or allergy is to consume milk, or a milk-derived product, on an empty stomach. If you have a problem with casein, the reaction will be fairly quick, within 15 to 30 minutes, and is usually in the form of burning, itchy eyes with a slight headache that will get more intense over time and last up to around two hours.

The solution for the above is simple avoid dairy and dairy-derived products.

Determining your Dairy Reaction

Make sure to read the labels of the foods you eat to ensure they are made from natural, whole milk. Incorporate them into your diet slowly to determine if you have a negative reaction to any individual product. Common negative reactions to dairy are sinus and lung congestion, asthma, bloating, gas and stomachaches. If you do have a reaction, it is important you stop consuming the offending product.

I find I can tolerate some dairy products, such as organic whole-milk cheeses, but have problems tolerating others, like cottage cheese and certain yogurts. Everyone is different; some people can't tolerate any dairy products while others can consume whatever they like without problems. The bottom line: Eat the highest quality dairy products and see what you do and don't have a reaction to.

THE DANGERS OF PROCESSED DAIRY PRODUCTS

There is one other little-discussed reason you may be intolerant to milk: Today's over-processed, pasteurized milk options are a far cry from what your great grandparents would have consumed. Your body may be able to tolerate natural, raw dairy, but react badly to the stuff at the supermarket. To understand why, we must go a few steps back to the source of the problem: the sad story of modern farm-raised cattle.

The Plight of Modern Cows

The modern cow is a freak of nature. Just a century ago, a cow produced two to three gallons of milk per day. Today's dairy cows produce up to four times this amount. This extraordinary output is the result of unnatural, high-protein diets and selective breeding that favors cows with abnormally active pituitary glands (the glands that produce milk-stimulating hormones and growth hormones). The controversial use of bovine growth hormones also helps to create more milk-productive cows.

The dire trade off, however, is that these unnatural hormones are passed to us through the processed milk. This comes at great cost. Excessive pituitary hormones are associated with tumor formation, so it's not surprising that some studies have linked milk consumption to cancer. On top of this, the modern cow is prone to many diseases due to its poor diet, and needs frequent doses of antibiotics to stay alive during its short life. These antibiotics also find their way into the milk supply—and thus your body—every time you drink milk from cows treated with such medications.

The quality of modern dairy products has been further compromised by the use of high-protein soybean meal as cow feed. Soy stimulates the production of large quantities of milk, but also causes a high rate of mastitis (i.e., breast inflammation typically caused by infection), sterility, liver problems and decreased longevity in cows. We have already discussed the dangers of soy in the human diet. However, not much is known about the effects of feeding high doses of soy to the animals we typically consume.

Nevertheless, since whatever an animal eats is stored in their muscle and fat tissues, we can reasonably assume that whatever they eat, we are effectively consuming in turn. Sadly, high-protein soy feed for livestock is becoming increasingly popular and is cheaper than feeding cattle what they should naturally consume: grass.

The meat from the animals fed a soy-based diet often comes with the seemingly healthy label of "vegetarian-fed." However that moniker can be very misleading, since many consumers naïve to the dangers of soy may mistakenly assume the term vegetarian-fed automatically makes the meat product a healthier choice. The best selection? Look for grass-fed meat instead.

A Grass-Fed Cow is a Healthy Cow

Cows are not designed to eat grains, corn and soy all the time, if at all. This type of diet makes them sick and is why cows on large-scale, commercial farms usually require large doses of antibiotics to remain well.

Cows are meant to eat grass. The rumen (the largest compartment of a cow's stomach) is where ingested grass is broken down by bacteria that naturally live in the cow's gut. These same bacteria are not, however, efficient at breaking down the grains, corn and soy products that the modern cow consumes today. Making matters worse, the corn and soy that is fed to most commercially farmed cows tends to be genetically modified (GMO). GMO products are controversial and generally considered to be unhealthy.

*This is a major reason why **free-range, grass-fed beef** is becoming increasingly popular. You are what you eat, but you also become what your food eats.*

The Problem with Pasteurization

Modern milk is progressively becoming more and more degraded. Besides concerns about the inferior conditions and inappropriate foods that the modern cow endures, various processing techniques further despoil today's milk. Perhaps the most egregious example of this is the use of pasteurization.

Pasteurization is a process in which raw milk is heated so as to destroy potentially illness-causing bacteria, molds and yeasts that may be present. Perhaps you were once taught that un-pasteurized milk contains harmful bacteria and is therefore dangerous to drink. What you probably weren't taught, however, is that the main reason today's milk has to be pasteurized is because of the modern cow's poor state of health.

The benefits of pasteurization and the safety of pasteurized dairy products have been greatly exaggerated. For example, all recent outbreaks of salmonella in milk occurred in pasteurized milk.

In contrast, raw milk contains lactic acid-producing bacteria that naturally protect against pathogens (disease-causing agents). Pasteurization destroys these helpful organisms, leaving the finished product devoid of any protective mechanism against harmful bacteria.

A 2009 study in the *Journal of Dairy Science* found that pasteurized milk, once refrigerated, became a safe haven for harmful bacteria. The study further found that raw milk (i.e., milk that was neither pasteurized nor homogenized) had low levels of harmful bacteria.

There are, sadly, even more problems with heat-treated milk products:

- The heat used in pasteurization damages several amino acids naturally found in milk (lysine and tyrosine). This makes it harder for humans to digest the proteins found in dairy.

- Pasteurization promotes the rancidity of unsaturated fatty acids, which can make milk go rancid more quickly.

- Overheating dairy destroys vitamins, alters lactose, and destroys the enzymes in milk that otherwise help the body to process and use the nutrients that milk contains, including calcium.

- Pasteurization prevents the absorption of vital nutrients into the small intestine and promotes the uptake of toxic substances.

All of this information isn't here to scare you off milk and dairy products. Rather, it is to inform you that your milk intolerance may be due to the processing of modern milk itself.

Going Raw

All of the healthy, milk-drinking populations studied by Dr. Weston Price consumed raw milk, raw cultured milk, or raw cheeses derived from healthy animals eating fresh grass or fodder. Happily, finding raw, whole milk and other products that originated from grass-fed cows is becoming increasingly convenient. Your local health food store will typically carry these products or know where you can purchase them.

To find the healthiest, highest quality raw milk in your area, I recommend finding a well-respected farmer in your area who follows safe and hygienic practices for their dairy cows. Not all raw milk is the same; its content is very dependent on the practices followed by individual farmers.

If you would like to try raw milk, first check out a raw dairy brand carried by your local natural foods market or health food store. These businesses usually have had long-term relationships with local farmers who grow and produce the products they sell, which eliminates the guesswork involved in finding a reputable raw-milk dairy.

Raw Cheese

Cheeses made from raw milk typically contain a full complement of enzymes. Because these enzymes can aid in the digestion of the cheese, they are more easily digested than cheeses made from pasteurized milk.

Cheese, in general, contains highly concentrated casein, which is well-tolerated by some but may have to be completely avoided by others. I'm a perfect example: I have a severe reaction to protein drinks comprising mainly casein, yet I can eat organic, whole-milk cheese without any problems.

A Special Caution for Immune-Compromised Populations

While healthy adults typically do very well with raw dairy products, the risk of getting sick from bacteria that may be present in raw milk is greater for infants and young children, the elderly, pregnant women, and people with weakened immune systems, such as people with cancer, an organ transplant or HIV/AIDS. For such immune-compromised populations, it's best to discuss the pros and cons of switching to raw milk with a medical practitioner before making the change.

THE PROCESSING OF FATS: WHY TO AVOID LOW-FAT DAIRY PRODUCTS

Another modern dairy processing method that makes me cringe is the removal of natural fats from dairy products. Simply put, I recommend that you avoid low-fat or reduced-fat dairy products; period. They are yet another example of a healthy product (natural, whole milk) being nutritionally neutered or even made unhealthy by modern processing techniques.

Low-fat milk is made by combining powdered milk and reduced-fat milk to prevent the final product from resembling milky water. To make powdered milk, regular milk is sprayed at high heat and pressure, which creates health-sapping oxidized cholesterol (which is not to be confused with the healthy, natural cholesterol we discussed earlier in this book). Therefore, when you consume reduced-fat milk or yogurt, thinking that it will help you avoid heart disease, you are actually consuming oxidized cholesterol which does the opposite.

Indeed, research has shown that oxidized cholesterol can *initiate* heart disease by causing plaque to build up in the arteries. In this way, low-fat dairy can actually speed up the development of heart disease that it claims to help prevent.

I typically avoid all low-fat and no-fat dairy products. They are usually packed full of chemicals or sugar in an effort to replace the texture and flavor of the natural and healthy fats that are removed for the sake of "diet food" marketing. They're just not worth it, and in fact may be inherently dangerous to our health.

Dairy of a Different Kind: Fermented Alternatives

The practice of fermenting or souring milk is found in almost all traditional herding cultures. Fermentation partially breaks down lactose and predigests casein, making fermented dairy products easier to digest. Common examples include yogurt and kefir (a yogurt-like dairy beverage).

Fermented dairy products are often well-tolerated by adults who can't comfortably drink milk. Similarly, butter and cream contain very little lactose and casein and are usually well-tolerated in their natural state, even by those who are lactose intolerant.

Individuals with an extreme intolerance for milk protein can eat butter in the form of ghee: clarified butter from which the milk solids have been removed. Ghee can be found in most health food stores.

Alternate Sources of Calcium

We have been brainwashed into believing that if we do not consume dairy products we will develop calcium deficiencies, which will impede the growth and continued strength of our bones. The truth is that, while dairy products are a great source of calcium, and while I believe dairy should be a part of your diet whenever feasible, milk products are not the only way to get the calcium you need.

Consider the case of mammals with some of the largest and most dense bones of any animal: elephants. Once an elephant is weaned from its mother's milk, it continues to grow and maintain solid bones that collectively weigh hundreds of pounds. How can an elephant do this without the calcium from its mother's milk? It instead gets calcium from dark green vegetation and grasses, the main staples of an adult elephant's diet.

Examples of healthy dark greens include dark-leafed salads, spinach, kale, broccoli and arugula. Moreover, these vegetables contain carotene and vitamins K1 and C. You get calcium, vitamins and fiber in one shot! Plus, a powerhouse of minerals is found in bones, so regularly preparing bone broths from chicken, beef or fish bones provides an abundant source of calcium, as well as many other minerals. Remember, a balanced diet is the best way to get most, if not all, of the nutrients you need to be healthy and strong.

MILK SUBSTITUTES

Today there is a wide variety of milk substitutes available for people who have a milk intolerance or allergy. If you can drink cow's milk, I highly recommend you do. Not only does full-fat, unprocessed milk contain vital fat and protein your body needs, but dairy products also help to add variety to your diet. If you cannot, or prefer not to, drink milk, there are some great alternatives.

Over the last several years, milk substitutes have become increasingly popular. Many people want to get their milk fix, minus any negative side effects that may occur due to dairy sensitivities and allergies, or from the hormones and antibiotics that are present in modern commercially produced milk.

If you drink an alternative milk product, be careful and read the label first. Some of these products are, unfortunately, loaded with sugars and additives. This is especially true of flavored milk substitutes, such as chocolate and vanilla varieties.

Soy Milk

In this section I discuss a number of alternatives to traditional dairy products. However, I have omitted the most popular of all milk substitutes: soy milk. Because of the soy-related health concerns previously outlined in Chapter 9, I do not recommend using soy milk as a dairy alternative whatsoever.

Comparing Milk and Non-Dairy Alternatives

I have included the nutritional information of the most popular milk substitutes below. These samples are from the most popular brand in each category, since these are the items you are most likely to see in your local grocery store. Make sure to read the label of the product you want to purchase, as ingredients and nutritional facts can change. This is meant to just be a guide to give you an idea of the dairy alternatives.

For comparison's sake, we'll first examine the nutritional content of 8 oz (1 cup) of whole cow's milk.

Whole Cow's Milk
Amounts listed are per 8 oz (1 cup)
146 calories
8 grams of fat
11 grams carbohydrates
13 grams of sugar (for those trying to lose weight, be careful in consuming too much milk due to its sugar content)
98 mg of sodium
0 grams of fiber
8 grams of protein

Contrast the above with the alternatives below. There is no perfect substitute; each has its own taste, benefits and weaknesses. It's best to just try a few and see which works best for you.

Almond Milk
Brand: Almond Breeze, Original (non-flavored)
Amounts listed are per 8 oz (1 cup)
60 calories
2.5 grams of fat
8 grams of carbs
7 grams of sugar
150 mg of sodium
1 gram of fiber
1 gram of protein

Hemp Milk
Brand: Rice Dream, Enriched Original
Amounts listed are per 8 oz (1 cup)

100 calories

6 grams of fat

9 grams of carbohydrates

6 grams of sugar

110 mg of sodium

0 grams of fiber

2 gram of protein

Rice Milk
Brand: Rice Dream, Enriched Original
Amounts listed are per 8 oz (1 cup)

120 calories

2.5 grams of fat

23 grams of carbohydrates

10 grams of sugar

100 mg of sodium

0 grams of fiber

1 gram of protein

Coconut Milk
Brand: SO Delicious, Original
Amounts listed are per 8 oz (1 cup)

80 calories

5 grams of fat

7 grams of carbohydrates

6 grams of sugars

15 mg of sodium

0 grams of fiber

1 gram of protein

10

Is Counting Calories Important?

You may now be wondering about how many calories you should eat, or whether you should be counting calories. Well, I don't believe in calorie counting, especially for the average person who is trying to lose weight.

Here's why: Calorie counting does not differentiate between healthy food and unhealthy food. It's just a numbers game. Let's say you are supposed to consume 2,000 calories per day in order to maintain a healthy body weight. Do you really think you will be healthy and maintain that ideal weight in the long term if you eat 2,000 calories of sugary, carbohydrate-rich foods instead of 2,000 calories of nutrient-rich fruits, vegetables and complete proteins each day? Or say you regularly consume 2,000 calories because you've been told that's what you must consume to be healthy and have a stable weight. Problem is, your day-to-day energy expenditures are going to be different, so there will be some days when you consume too few calories and others when you consume too many. Wouldn't it make more sense to eat healthy foods only when you are hungry, and to not try to play an unrealistic numbers counting game?

Maintaining a healthy weight and lifestyle involves many factors besides the amount of calories you consume. Consider the case of someone who starves himself or herself throughout the day in order to have a high-sugar, high-calorie latte and pastry in the afternoon. This clearly is not the road to all-day energy and well-being. Yet this is the type of behavior that continually stems from calorie-counting diets. The time and energy you waste on counting calories can (and I argue, should) be invested into something more productive in your life.

Although I do not advocate calorie counting, it's still important for you to understand how calories relate to fad diet programs and weight loss. An understanding of calories can be a useful tool; herein we'll discuss how this can best be used in your quest for health and weight loss.

CALORIES DEFINED

Calories are units of energy. More specifically, a calorie is the amount of energy (in the form of heat) that it takes to raise the temperature of one gram of water by one degree Celsius (1.8 degrees Fahrenheit).

Here's the macronutrient-to-calorie breakdown:
1 gram of protein = 4 calories
1 gram of carbohydrate = 4 calories
1 gram of fat = 9 calories

When is a Calorie Not a Calorie?

However, the calories listed on food packages are technically measured in kilocalories or kcal (1000 calories = one kilocalorie). When we discuss the calories of foods, it is an understood convention that "calories" refers to kcals. For this reason, kcals can also sometimes be referred to as *food calories* or *dietary calories.*

It definitely looks better to the consumer to see that he or she is consuming 100 calories (actually 100 kcal) instead of 100,000 calories. (Isn't it interesting to learn how we are duped right from the beginning when it comes to defining calories?) For the sake of simplicity, I'll stick to the conventional use of caloric measures used on food labels today and refer to one kilocalorie in layman's terms as one calorie.

ENERGY IN VS. ENERGY OUT: THE FIRST LAW OF THERMODYNAMICS

The number of calories in a food is a measure of how much potential energy that food possesses. A gram of carbohydrate contains four calories of energy, a gram of protein contains four calories, and a gram of fat contains nine calories.

Here's where it gets interesting: Today's fad diets are primarily based on the **first law of thermodynamics**, which states that energy can be changed from one form to another but cannot be created or destroyed. In scientific terms, this means that the change in the internal energy of a system is equal to the amount of heat (energy) supplied to the system, minus the amount of work performed (also in terms of energy) by the system on its surroundings.

The first law of thermodynamics, when applied to weight gain or loss, is expressed as **calories in versus calories out**. That is, energy you eat versus energy you expend in everyday activities and in just keeping your bodily systems alive and functioning all day and night. This principle means that if you consume more calories (energy) than you expend, you will gain weight. This is because unused calories will be stored, typically as fat tissue.

Conversely, if you use more energy than you consume in calories in a given time period, you will lose weight. This is because your body will make up for your caloric (energy) shortfall by retrieving stored forms of energy in your fat tissues. This, in theory, is what is responsible for decreasing your dress size. But let's examine why this may not work out so precisely in practice.

Theoretical Accuracy in Caloric Measures

One pound of body fat contains roughly 3,500 calories of energy. Let's say you consumed 25 calories more than you expended, every day, for one year. According to the first law of thermodynamics, you would gain a little over 2.6 pounds of body fat annually (25 calories per day, times 365 days in a year, divided by the 3,500 calories in a pound of fat equals 2.6 pounds of body fat).

So what do 25 additional calories in your diet look like? Here are some of the items that contain 25 calories: less than half an apple, a small bite of a cookie, a bite of a banana or one raw tomato. So, according to the calories-in-versus-calories-out theory, you will gain 2.6 pounds of fat in one year if you have a small bite of a cookie or eat one tomato beyond your required daily calorie intake.

I don't know about you, but to me this just doesn't add up in the practical, real world we live in. Why not?

Our bodies (and not hypothetical calorie counts) are the final determiner on how these units of energy are used or broken down. Everyone has a different metabolic rate (the efficiency by which food is broken down for energy). Outside of having access to complex equipment in a physiology research lab, you cannot know your resting metabolic rate with 100 percent accuracy. The calories your body should use in one day—as listed in diet books and internet sites—can only ever be an *estimation*, typically based on your age and gender. There is no real-world way to know the true, exact amount of daily calories your body requires. As with all physiological traits, everyone is very different in this regard.

Acknowledged Errors in Physiological Measurements

The measurement of human function and physiological processes (such as your exact temperature or metabolic rate) is limited by numerous practical and theoretical factors. As can your body temperature, your metabolic rate can fluctuate quite a bit based on lifestyle and environmental factors.

Even top scientists with complex lab equipment have to make certain theoretical assumptions (which may or may not be accurate) to measure biological markers. This produces known sources and ranges of error in any scientific measurement of human physiology.

Simple Life Health Point: Mass-produced charts about physiological targets such as caloric intake or maximum heart rates—while good estimations—can never be 100 percent accurate when it comes to the unique nuances of how your body works. Where calories are concerned, worry about quality before quantity.

How does this apply to your weight loss? Although resting metabolic rate charts exist for different age, weight and gender groups, no chart can tell you the precise metabolic rate that exists in your unique body, in your unique circumstance. In short, there is no way to know the exact "magic number" of calories you should eat every day for absolute energy balance. You may be able to come to a pretty good estimate, but that's as close as you can get. This means the calories-in-versus-calories-out equation, while helpful as a general guideline, is **not** something to be religiously followed as the only answer to your weight loss equation.

Calorie counting, in real life and outside of a research lab, is far from an exact science. Our bodies, when fed natural healthy foods, will determine energy-in-versus-energy-out regulation through various chemical processes. I don't eat the same amount of calories every day and my weight is almost always within one to two percent of its normal range. This is primarily due to consistency in my diet and exercise habits: I eat healthy, natural foods when I'm actually hungry. There are no gimmicks and no tricks on the road to health!

DIFFERENT BODIES, DIFFERENT REACTIONS

Remember, no two bodies react in the same way to eating the same amount of calories. Hormones and enzymes also control how much fat we store—it's not just about the calories. Plus, refined carbohydrates are the main catalyst behind the fat-storage process.

How can we know that fat storage is hormonally controlled? Consider the contrast between the body shapes of men versus women. If the calories-in-versus-calories-out dogma was absolutely true and independent of any other factors, then the body shapes of both men and women would be almost identical! Yet men mainly store fat around their waists, and women mainly store fat around their hips, rear and thighs. This indicates that it's not only the quantity of calories consumed that controls fat storage, but also confirms that hormones and metabolism mainly control where and how much fat storage will occur.

Drastically cutting calories rarely leads to a healthier and leaner body. The body responds to large caloric deficiencies (when you burn more energy than you consume) by reducing the release and production of fat-burning enzymes. At the same time, your body increases its release of fat-storing enzymes. Once this happens, your body alters its hormonal output to slow your metabolic rate because it essentially thinks it is starving when faced with extreme calorie restrictions.

It is, therefore, a dieter's mistake to continue to eat nutrient-empty processed foods and solely focus on reducing the overall number of calories consumed. Instead, he or she should concentrate on consuming nutrient-dense, natural foods until comfortably satisfied. If you consume a nutritionally deficient diet and then cut calories (quantity) instead of improving the quality of foods you eat, you will only become even more nutrient-deficient, and your body's intuitive suspicion that it's starving will become fact!

Simple Life Health Point: The longer you eat insufficient calories, the slower your metabolism becomes and the more sluggish and unhealthy you feel. This is why starvation diets never work in the long term. You must eat well to be well!

Caloric Quality versus Quantity

One thing is clear when it comes to calories: Natural foods almost always have far fewer calories than highly processed foods of equal (or more likely, of inferior) nutritional value. For example, one serving of nacho cheese Doritos (which is merely one ounce of chips) contains 140 calories. You would have to consume almost a pound of raw carrots in order to consume this amount of total calories.

People eating a 2,000-calorie-per-day diet would only have to eat 11 ounces of Doritos to meet their calorie quota, but they could have eaten 8 pounds of carrots in order to receive the same caloric result. Plus, I'm fairly confident there is no argument anywhere that says Doritos are nutritionally superior to carrots. **Quality over quantity is key.**

Moreover, why consume your thoughts with *calories* every second of the day? "How many calories have I eaten today?" "How many more calories do I have left to eat today?" "Oops, I exceeded my calories for the day and it's not even 4 p.m. . . . I guess I won't eat tonight!"

I know of these thoughts firsthand because I've been a victim of the calorie theory myself.

Simple Life Health Point: Counting calories is tiresome and time-consuming. Instead, worry about the quality of your food and invest the rest of your time in something much more enjoyable.

The good news is that you don't really need to count calories in order to be healthy! Some people love numbers, so if you do want to count calories there is nothing wrong with that approach, as long as those calories are coming from healthy foods. You just have to remember it is not an exact science.

11

Your Body Is an Ocean— Understanding Proper Water and Salt Consumption

Water makes up nearly 60 percent of your body weight, and two-thirds of that water is contained inside your cells. It's estimated that 75 percent of Americans are chronically dehydrated. Here's why, and how to avoid falling into that harmful category.

WATER'S MANY BENEFITS

In the human body, water has many functions. For example, it acts as a solvent, a catalyst, a lubricant, a temperature regulator and a mineral source. It helps flush toxins out of your system and cleanses your kidneys—all-important aspects of your body's healing processes.

Water's contribution to health is often overlooked, yet it's one of the easiest and cheapest deficiencies to correct. Here are some helpful facts about water:

- Ever crave a 3 p.m. pick-me-up? The solution may be simple: A lack of water is the number one trigger of daytime fatigue.

- Preliminary research indicates that drinking eight to ten cups of water per day is capable of significantly easing joint and back pain for up to 80 percent of sufferers.

- A mere two percent drop in the amount of water in your body can trigger short-term memory challenges with basic math problems and difficulties focusing on a computer screen or printed page.

- Drinking five glasses of water daily decreases the risk of colon cancer by 45 percent, slashes the risk of breast cancer by 79 percent, and cuts the likelihood of developing bladder cancer by 50 percent.

- Water is free. Unlike carbonated soft drinks, which can cost $1.50 per bottle, tap water costs you nothing. If you nix your daily soft drink habit and drink filtered tap water, you could save $550 or more per year!

- Water helps prevent bladder infections. Studies indicate that men who consume more than 10 glasses of water per day are less likely to develop bladder infections than those who do not.

- Water promotes cardiac health.

HOW MUCH WATER SHOULD I BE DRINKING?

According to most sources, your daily water intake should be about 12 cups of water (96 ounces) per day. This doesn't mean you should force down a jug of water right now. Instead, on average you'll consume four cups of water (32 ounces) through the water-rich foods you eat (such as fruits and vegetables). This leaves eight cups (64 ounces) that must come from fluid intake.

Consider our prehistoric cousins: Would they have been able to consume 64 ounces of water outside of what was already contained in their everyday foods on a consistent basis? Maybe, but maybe not! They certainly didn't have the same convenient drinking options that we have.

Here's the easiest way I have found to roughly estimate the ideal amount of daily water to consume: Divide your weight in half and then drink that number in ounces of water. For example, if you weigh 150 pounds you need 75 ounces of water (which includes the water content of the foods you eat) each day. Obviously, this is less than the recommended "textbook" amount previously stated. However, I recommend using the weight-based guide since it's less generic and more individual-specific.

Be cautious not to drink too much water; a range of five to eight cups per day should be sufficient. Of course, on days that you're more physically active you'll need to consume additional fluids and salt (since salt is also lost through sweat) to maintain proper hydration and electrolyte balance.

How can you tell if you need to drink more water? Your urine will be dark yellow and smelly. If you're properly hydrated, your urine will be pale and practically odorless.

There's one exception to this observation: If you take a daily multi-vitamin, your urine will appear bright yellow and have a strong odor in the hours after you take it, since your body excretes any vitamins and minerals it doesn't need. This is normal, and your urine will become clear if you're properly hydrated as the day continues.

Other common symptoms of dehydration include constipation,

dry and itchy skin, acne, nosebleeds, repeated urinary tract infections, dry and unproductive coughs, constant sneezing, sinus pressure and headaches. If you suffer from one or more of these concerns, drink more water and see if that alleviates the problem.

WATER AND DIGESTION

Some research has shown that consuming excess liquids with meals dilutes stomach acid and puts undue strain on digestive processes. I recommend you avoid drinking too much liquid before or after a meal, and sip beverages slowly with meals. Drinking ice-cold water also makes digestion very difficult. Avoid adding ice to your beverages; drink them at room temperature whenever possible.

I usually don't drink any liquids with my meals. And if I do, I only take a couple of sips. Since doing so, I've noticed a drastic improvement in the quality of my digestion, and I rarely feel any bloating or discomfort after a meal. If you're used to drinking a lot of liquids with meals, try to gradually reduce the amounts you drink with food over time and see if you notice a difference.

WATER ON THE GO

The best way to make sure you get enough water throughout the day is to carry a stainless steel or glass reusable water bottle everywhere you go. (Avoid aluminum bottles; unlike steel, aluminum is a reactive metal. Translation? It can leach toxins into your water.) I have kept a bottle of water near me for years. Remember, you'll drink more water when it's handy and convenient, so set yourself up for success!

A reusable bottle is also far more environmentally friendly than plastic throwaway bottles. Plus, plastic bottles have been shown to leach Bisphenol A (BPA). This toxic chemical is an endocrine (hormonal system) disruptor. BPA can mimic the body's own hormones (primarily estrogen) and may lead to negative health effects. Even BPA-free plastic water bottles can have chemicals that can be harmful to us, so I definitely recommend going with the stainless steel or glass options I mentioned above.

SALT IS NOT THE PROBLEM

Too much food-based fructose causes high blood pressure, not salt, recent research reveals. This is a far cry from what you've probably heard about why so many Americans develop heart disease and hypertension (high blood pressure).

Probably the most telling fact is that we consume about fifty percent less salt today than we did before refrigeration. Before refrigeration, foods were primarily cured (preserved) by using natural salt. Considering hypertension was almost unheard of before refrigeration, it just flat-out doesn't make sense that salt consumption is a primary cause of hypertension today.

Sadly, instead of targeting our real dietary concerns (highly processed carbohydrates, especially those that contain fructose) we've been eliminating salt from our diets, causing even worse health problems than we originally started with.

Why? Salt is a vital dietary nutrient and very healthy when consumed in moderation. To wit, entirely eliminating salt from your meals may have detrimental health consequences.

This begs the question: What's the right way to eat this essential, yet much-maligned, mineral? The key is to know the right quantity and quality of salt to include in your new way of eating.

Most people believe that salt is just salt. However, there's a big difference between table salt (refined sodium chloride) and natural salt, such as sea salt. While table salt damages your health, natural salt has healing properties and is beneficial to consume. It's that simple.

The Dangers of Table Salt

Natural salt is made up of around 84 percent sodium chloride (the main mineral constituent of salt). In contrast, table salt is 98 percent sodium chloride. The remaining 16 percent of natural salt is composed of naturally occurring minerals. The remaining two percent of table salt consists of man-made chemicals—many of which are unhealthy.

Some of the negative consequences of eating table (i.e. refined) salt are:

- It increases perspiration and decreases muscle contractility (i.e., ability of the muscle to contract), including in the heart muscle.

- It acidifies the blood, which can cause liver and heart problems, rheumatism and gastric ulcers.

- It creates arrhythmias (inconsistent heart rhythms) from its abnormal impact on nerves, and hardens arteries and other tissues. It also fosters calcium and fatty deposits on artery walls.

- It inhibits digestion, damages and depletes enzymes, upsets the body's sodium/potassium balance, and creates an acidic stomach.

- It over-stimulates the nervous system by activating the adrenal glands.

- It puts a huge burden on the kidneys and can weaken them until they can no longer function.

Refined salt starts out as natural salt. However, its chemical structure is altered when it's dried at 1,200 degrees Fahrenheit. This process mainly leaves sodium chloride molecules behind, since most of the minerals found in natural salt are basically baked off. Next, anti-caking and flow agents are added, which prevent the salt crystals from clumping together. Unfortunately, some of these chemicals are dangerous and unhealthy.

These may include the following:

Sodium ferrocyanide is an anti-caking agent found in common table salt. It's also used in:

- Pigment production

- Street and snow removal salts (as an anti-caking agent)

- The chemical separation of trace metallic ions (for use in various chemical processes)

- Cleaning agents

- Corrosion inhibitors

- Steel surface treatment

- Galvanization processes (e.g., of silver and pewter)

- Photographic development processes

- The fermentation of citric acid and ascorbic acid

Sodium aluminosilicate is another anti-caking agent used in table salt. It has a high brightness and relatively coarse particle size and can partially replace titanium oxide in latex paints as a flattening agent. In addition, some dry laundry detergents, as well as powdered carpet and room deodorizers, contain sodium aluminosilicate as a flow agent. Aluminum-based chemicals, including sodium aluminosilicate, have also been linked to heavy metal toxicity and possibly Alzheimer's disease.

Other chemicals added to refined salt include **sodium silicoaluminate**, which is thought to be associated with kidney problems and mineral malabsorption. **Sodium acetate**, another added chemical, may cause elevated blood pressure, kidney disturbances and water retention.

The Right Sources of Salt

The best way to make sure you're getting enough sodium in your diet is to eat a healthy diet with very little or no processed foods, and add salt to taste.

Research indicates that sea salt in moderation (between one-and-a-half and two-and-a-half teaspoons per day) is healthy. Of course, this is in conjunction with a nutritious diet with very few processed foods and few carbohydrates.

Sea salt has many natural healing properties and plays an important role in your body's healthy physiology.

Natural salt replaces lost electrolytes and helps to balance the body's pH level (a measure of the body's relative acidity or alkalinity such as exists in the blood). It helps to stimulate the liver, helps regulate muscle contractions (mainly of the heart), and stimulates the production of digestive acids. Salt is also effective in stabilizing irregular heartbeats, and the iodine it contains is crucial to the thyroid gland.

Salt is vital for balancing sugar levels in the blood. It's also necessary for the absorption of food particles through the intestinal tract, for clearing mucus plugs and sticky phlegm out of the lungs (particularly for sufferers of lung conditions such as asthma and cystic fibrosis), for clearing up sinus congestion and catarrh (excess mucus secretions of the sinuses), and for the prevention of muscle cramps, gout and gouty arthritis, and varicose veins and spider veins on the legs and thighs. The benefits of sea salt go on and on.

Happily, the last few years have seen a rise in the prevalence of food products containing sea salt instead of refined salt. Make sure to read product labels to find out what's in your favorite foods.

The two best natural salts to use are Celtic sea salt and Himalayan crystal salt. These natural salts are some of the most pure and minimally processed in the world. They also taste fantastic—far better than refined table salt. Fortunately, minimally processed sea salt and safely mined Himalayan salt are becoming more readily available.

A final word of caution: There are now several salt substitutes available to consumers. Generally, salt-like replacements should be avoided since they're made of unhealthy chemicals. Remember, sea salt is the best and most natural way to get proper amounts of sodium and other minerals.

If you don't have medical clearance to use even natural sea salt in your diet, choose health-boosting spices or dried herbs for a food flavor kick before turning to chemically based pseudo-salt products (think garlic granules, fresh ground pepper or dried oregano to start).

EATING FOR EXERCISE: SALT AND SPORTS

Now that you're working out, you may be tempted to reach for a sports drink to replenish your fluids and, as the marketing teams behind bottled beverages are quick to claim, your electrolytes (more on these molecules below). Please don't—that gulp of Gatorade or its neon-colored clone may seriously set you back, both financially and health-wise. Here's why.

Your bodily fluids are salty, including your blood, plasma and interstitial fluid (the fluid between your cells). Each has a high concentration of sodium chloride.

When you exercise, you lose minerals such as sodium, magnesium and potassium, which are types of electrolytes (salts with certain chemical properties in common).

Electrolytes are what your cells—especially your nerve, heart and muscle cells—use to carry electrical impulses (nerve impulses and muscle contractions). These allow messages (sensorial input) to travel from one part of the body to another.

Your kidneys work to keep the electrolyte concentration in your blood constant. These electrolytes must be replaced through dietary sources.

This brings us to sodium, which is one such electrolyte, and an important one at that. If your blood sodium levels drop below an ideal range (a condition known as *hyponatremia*), your body's fluid levels rise and your cells begin to swell. Hyponatremia has come into the public eye because marathon runners have died from not replacing the sodium lost during sporting events by drinking only plain water.

This is why most sports drinks have sodium chloride or potassium chloride added to them (not to mention a great deal of sugar, which should be avoided). Although sports drinks contain electrolytes, they don't contain anywhere near enough to replenish your body's supply. Moreover, the electrolytes they *do* contain are usually from synthetic sources and not from natural vitamins and minerals. Meaning? What they do is drain you of your health and hard-earned money, as the following story illustrates.

Not long ago, I saw an aspiring young sportsman in the local grocery store who filled his cart with about 20 bottles of a popular sports drink. I asked him why he had so many. He said he had been working out a lot, trying to make the high school football team, and needed to replace his electrolytes.

When I asked him *why* he needed to replace his electrolytes, he didn't know—it seemed he had simply picked up the idea from one of those popular sports drink commercials. I grabbed one of the bottles and showed him how much sugar was in his sports drink (20 grams!) and indicated that I had a better solution.

I explained that electrolytes are found in sea salt and are important for muscle contractions; therefore, they're very important for athletes to replace. Then I led him to the sea salt section of the store and told him that for a couple of bucks he could have all the electrolytes he needed. He could simply add a pinch or two of salt to plain water to make his own sports drink, and a much healthier one at that. He was very thankful and just shook his head as he put back all of the sugary sports drinks. I encourage you to do the same.

I wish I had had had this information when I was a young athlete. It would have saved me a lot of money on sports drinks and helped me take better care of my health. Sometimes simple is best.

12

Sleep Yourself to Health

So many of us go through the day feeling tired. It's no wonder: In the past 40 years, adult Americans have reduced the amount of time they sleep each night by two hours! A recent survey found that many people sleep less than six hours per night, yet most researchers agree that adults need seven to nine hours of nightly slumber.

Sleeping patterns appear to have some correlation to body weight: As sleep time decreases, average weight increases. In 1960, only one in nine adults was obese. Today that number has jumped to nearly one in three.

Sleep difficulties occur in 75 percent of us at least a few nights per week and a short-lived bout of insomnia is generally nothing to worry about. However, chronic sleep deprivation is a bigger concern, since it can lead to weight gain, high blood pressure and a lowered immunity to illnesses.

Some useful sleep facts:

- **Learning and memory:** Sleep allows the brain to commit new information to memory through a process called memory consolidation. In studies, people who slept after learning a task did better on subsequent tests.

- **Metabolism and weight:** Chronic sleep deprivation may cause weight gain by affecting the way our bodies process and store carbohydrates, and by altering levels of hormones that affect appetite.

- **Safety:** Chronic fatigue can lead to daytime drowsiness and unintentional naps. Such episodes may cause falls and potentially deadly mishaps, such as medical errors and air traffic and road accidents.

- **Mood:** Sleep loss may result in irritability, impatience, an inability to concentrate and moodiness. Too little sleep can also leave you too tired to do the things you enjoy.

- **Cardiovascular health:** Serious sleep disorders have been linked to hypertension, increased levels of stress hormones and irregular heart rhythms.

- **Disease:** Sleep deprivation alters immune function, including the activity of "killer" immune cells (the "soldiers" of your immune system that seek out and destroy threatening viruses and bacteria that have invaded your body). Good sleep habits may also help fight cancer.

I know with our busy schedules, families and other obligations, it's often difficult to get seven to nine hours of sleep per night. But sleep goes such a long way toward improving your health and body shape that I urge you to try, even if you can only add a little bit of time to your nightly rest.

Before industrialized society existed, our activity and sleep patterns were very in tune with the cycles of the sun and our natural environment. Because of this long history, when light stimulates your skin or eyes, *regardless of the source*, your brain and hormonal system think it's morning.

CIRCADIAN RHYTHMS

Your natural, or *circadian*, rhythm is the internal body clock that regulates the roughly 24-hour cycle of biological processes shared by animals and plants alike. If we were to follow our natural circadian rhythms, we would start winding down as the sun set and would be ready for sleep around 10 p.m. Most physical repairs occur while sleeping between 10 p.m. and 2 a.m. After 2 a.m., and until you wake up at sunlight, your body is more focused on psychogenic (mental) repair.

Understanding how your body reacts to light is critical, especially in a day and age when we watch TV or play with smart phones in brightly lit rooms well past when the sun has gone down. In response to this light, artificial or otherwise, your hormonal system releases the stress hormone cortisol. This is because your body considers light to be a form of electromagnetic stress, and cortisol readies your body for activity and the start of the day.

Normal cortisol levels peak between 6 a.m. and 9 a.m. At the end of the day, when darkness falls, your cortisol levels are greatly reduced. At the same time, melatonin (a sleep-regulating hormone) is released, as are growth and repair hormones. The take-home message? Use light to wake up, and dim the lights (including smart phone, computer and TV screens) well before you want to fall asleep.

Studies have shown that people who have chaotic, irregular sleep schedules tend to release excessive amounts of cortisol throughout the day. If you're one of them, you may consequently suffer from fatigue of the adrenal glands (which are responsible for fight-or-flight responses). Adrenal gland fatigue causes additional storage of stomach fat, thus contributing to obesity. As if you needed another reason to catch some zzz's!

You may, however, be concerned about oversleeping. To ensure you rise at a consistent time every morning, leave your window blinds open. This allows natural sunlight to enter your room, stimulating the production of cortisol and gradually waking your body.

This may be impractical if you live in an urban setting where streetlights are on all night and can disturb the quality of your sleep. Consistency in your sleep patterns will usually ensure that you naturally wake at the same time in the mornings, or you can purchase a clock that gently wakes you by simulating the gradual increase in light of sunrise. This is much more pleasant to wake to than a jarring alarm!

SIMPLE TIPS FOR A GOOD NIGHT'S REST

1. Reduce or eliminate your exposure to bright lights, such as fluorescent lights, for at least two hours before you go to bed.

2. Go to sleep by 10:30 p.m. This means you need to be in bed by 10 p.m. to allow enough time to wind down and fall asleep.

3. Don't consume any products or drinks containing sugar, caffeine or nicotine after 1:00 in the afternoon. This will

allow your body sufficient time to eliminate most or all of these non-sleep-friendly stimulants before you snooze.

4. Get some exercise every day. However, try not to exercise too close to bedtime. I recommend completing your workout at least two hours before you head to bed.

5. Make sure you've finished your last meal of the day at least three hours before you retire. A light supper will be easier to digest and keep you more comfortable as you prepare for sleep.

6. Make sure your room is as dark as possible during the night. If it's difficult or impossible to make your room dark, a sleep mask can be invaluable.

7. To prevent sleep-disrupting bathroom visits, don't drink any liquids two hours before bedtime.

8. Try reading an inspirational book 30 to 45 minutes before bedtime (no detective novels, however!).

9. Follow your body's natural rhythms. I know my body won't go to sleep if it's not ready. If I force myself to try to sleep when I'm not yet tired, I just remain awake for longer than if I had stayed up until I was ready to fall asleep naturally.

10. Follow a regular sleep schedule. You should go to bed and wake up at the same time every day whenever possible. I aim to do this even on weekends and holidays so I don't have to readjust my sleep cycle when the weekend or holiday is over. When I sleep on a consistent schedule, I have a noticeable boost in my everyday energy levels and experience fewer sleepless or restless nights.

13

Stress—the Silent Killer

It's no secret that in today's hectic world we're continuously bombarded by stress. Heck, that's where *The Simple Life* concept came from: I want to help people live a simpler, happier and healthier life. I know, throughout my journey, I've dealt with the same daily stresses that most people today deal with, resulting in some pretty serious negative health consequences. Realizing we're stressed out is the easy part, though; the more challenging part is figuring out what to do about it.

What I'm referring to when I'm talking about life stress is *chronic* stress. Intermittent stress is something that all organisms deal with, even plants, and it's perfectly normal and short-lived. This type of stress helps organisms adapt to their environment in order to thrive. When under chronic stress, however, you will experience some or all of the following:

Increased heart rate, blood flow, and oxygen intake by your lungs. Parts of your immune system becoming temporarily suppressed, which negatively affects your inflammatory response to disease and pathogens.

As our stress levels continue to increase, the health world is realizing the many afflictions and diseases that can be attributed to this silent killer.

Here are the top 10:

- Accelerated aging

- Asthma

- Alzheimer's disease

- Chronic headaches and migraines

- Depression

- Diabetes

- Digestive issues

- Heart disease

- Obesity/chronic weight gain

- Premature death

As you can see, this is pretty much the laundry list of health problems and diseases that most people suffer from today.

Here's a key point for those trying to lose weight: Chronic stress will wreak havoc with the hormone cortisol, which causes your body to store fat and inhibits it from burning it for energy.

I can't make this any clearer—even if you follow every piece of healthy living advice outlined in this book, you'll never reach your optimal health potential if you don't reduce your stress levels. That's how detrimental chronic stress is to your mental and physiological well-being.

This chapter is going to be short and sweet, as most people realize they have too much stress in their lives, and I would say most also know it's having a negative impact on their health. So instead of going into some long-winded diatribe about stress and disease, I'm going to give you the nitty gritty of what I use, and have used, with clients over the years to reduce stress. If there's one main key concept you can take from my *Simple Life* series, even though I delve into a multitude of topics, it's the reduction of the stresses we're bombarded with today.

Here's my Top 5 list of stress reducers:

1. Exercise. I can't tell you how important exercise is in dealing with stress. I've used exercise as my decompression and getaway from it all for decades. Not only do I improve my health and physique, I also manage my stress levels. I can't say it enough—regular exercise *has* to be an integral part of your healthy lifestyle plan.

2. Get Your Finances in Order. When I ask my clients what their biggest stressor is, they almost always say **money**. It's no surprise that we're stressed out by money, considering the "consumer nation" society we live in today. If you implement a good exercise program and get your finances in order, I will guarantee your stress levels will be greatly reduced. (Be on the lookout for an entire *Simple Life* book on financial freedom in the near future.)

3. Fire Bad Friends and Family Members. Yep, a little tough love here. Trust me, I had to learn this one the hard way. Some people are just detrimental to your life; period, I like to call them "takers," because all they do is take up all your free time and increase your stress by their inability to manage their lives. The worst part is, most of their drama is self-created. Instead of dealing with it themselves, they use the people around them, making their lives miserable as well. I have heard, "But they're family" too many times to count. It doesn't matter—crappy people are crappy people, even if you're related to them. Disconnect from them and move on.

4. Surround Yourself With Like-Minded People. I touch on this a bit in the exercise chapter later in this book. Not only have my stress levels been greatly reduced by surrounding myself with people who are interested in the same lifestyle as myself, but this has also benefited me as an entrepreneur. By being around other entrepreneurs trying to simplify their lives, I've learned more than I could have ever imagined. You want to get in shape? Surround yourself with people who want the same thing or are already in shape. Want to be a writer? Surround yourself with writers!

5. Meditate Daily. OK, I know I may have lost a couple of you here; I don't necessarily mean going into some out-of-body state (though if you can do that, that's awesome!). What I mean is spending 5 to 10 minutes a day in a peaceful space with your eyes closed and quieting your mind. I like doing this in the sauna at the gym when no one is around, and I will tell you I feel fantastic afterward.

If you can't manage your stress with any of these techniques, or you feel completely overwhelmed, you need to get professional help. I don't say this lightly; there are mental health professionals for a reason. Forget any of the stigmas associated with seeing a mental health professional—this is about your health and well-being. Despite what anyone else might think, you need to do all you can to make sure you achieve a healthy and happy life.

14

You've Gotta Move! Exercise 101

What you eat plays an enormous role in your vitality and physical appearance. While the importance of nutritious, natural eating habits cannot be understated, it's also important to get moving.

I'd love to see you in the gym regularly. But before you bemoan the idea, know that a major part of any fitness-oriented lifestyle is not just the sweat you generate in the gym. It's how much you move all day long.

What do I mean by this? Consider the world that humans evolved in: a primal world without cars or modern appliances ... or gyms.

It's estimated that prehistoric hunter-gatherers expended three to five times the amount of energy we do every day, all while consuming far fewer, if any, empty calories (they did consume much healthier calories than we do today to fuel their activities). Yet they would not spend three or four hours in a gym during the week. Obviously—there were no fitness centers! The physical activities they performed would have been of short duration and high intensity, unless they were traveling for long distances.

How would our prehistoric brethren get their exercise? Their sport was life itself: hunting, gathering, building and maintaining shelter, and basic survival activities such as sprinting away from a predator.

In our modern world, we can get away with moving a woefully insignificant amount. Indeed, it's possible to be financially successful and barely move one's body whatsoever in our day and age. But it's just common sense that walking a few hundred steps per day is not enough to keep you lean and healthy! Our bodies function best in conjunction with a lifestyle that involves relatively constant movement all day (*primal* movement). Yet many of us go from home to a car to a work desk to a car to home to the couch, to watch other people play sports on television.

So what's the solution? It's *Simple Life* movement, which is encompassed in two steps.

First, look for ways to be more active throughout the day. This is the non-gym stuff, and you already know about it: Take the stairs instead of the elevator. Park further away from the store. Go for a 10-minute walk around your workplace instead of drinking another soda or coffee. Walk to your colleague's desk at the office to talk instead of sending another email. Little movements, all day long, add up over time. That's the first part of *The Simple Life* movement concept.

Second, you need to start a regular exercise program. Don't worry if you've never even thought about joining a gym before. Here's all the information you need to be well-informed and comfortable when starting an exercise program.

SECRETS TO A SUCCESSFUL WORKOUT

An effective and healthy workout has several components. They include a warm-up, some stretching, cardio training, resistance training and a cool-down.

I don't want you wasting your workout time on ineffective exercise! This section will enable you to take charge of your exercise habits with confidence and get better results without squandering your precious time.

We'll begin by describing some principles of exercise that will help you with your new routine.

Categories of Exercise

All exercise can be categorized as either *aerobic* (meaning with oxygen) or *anaerobic* (without oxygen).

Aerobic training refers to a type of longer-term energy use in the body that requires the presence of oxygen molecules. Examples include jogging, walking, moderate bike riding and aerobics classes (now you know where the name came from). Aerobic exercise also activates your immune system, helps your heart pump blood more efficiently, and increases your stamina over time.

If you're new to exercise, you may not know what they mean down at the gym when they refer to the cardio machines or cardio classes. Basically, *cardio* is aerobic exercise that elevates your heart rate and makes you sweat—think running, dancing or cycling. It strengthens your cardiovascular system (your heart and blood vessels), hence its everyday nickname, cardio.

Anaerobic training is a type of short-term energy use in the body that does not require the presence of oxygen molecules. Shot putting, pitching, weightlifting and powerlifting are all examples of anaerobic activities. This type of training makes you stronger, creates denser muscle tissue, and increases the efficiency with which your body burns energy (increases your metabolism).

Aerobic and anaerobic exercises may be further organized into these categories:

Interval training can be a combination of aerobic and anaerobic training. You perform this type of training by alternating short bursts of high-intensity exercise with gentle recovery periods. Riding a stationary bike can be an example, if you go for a burst of all-out, high-intensity pedaling for 30 seconds, trying to reach 80 percent of your maximum heart rate (this is described in more detail below). This would then be followed by 30 to 90 seconds (depending on your current physical condition) of easy riding, bringing your heart rate back down. The sequence would then repeat. I usually do this routine for only twenty minutes (including my warm-up) before I'm shot! I can assure you that people looking to push themselves will find this is an excellent training method.

Strength training (also known as **resistance** or **weight training**) is a one- to four-set training routine, depending on your exercise experience, performing enough repetitions to exhaust your muscles. The weight you use should be heavy enough so that you can only perform a maximum of 12 repetitions, but no fewer than four repetitions. I recommend you continue to advance in your exercise program until you are performing some type of resistance training two to three times a week. You can also perform strength training with almost any resistance-based exercise and it's an excellent choice when you only have a short amount of time to squeeze in a workout.

Core exercises target the 29 core muscles that are primarily located in your abdomen, back and pelvis. These muscles are the foundation for movement and support for your entire body. Core exercises—such as crunches, planks and back extensions—help improve your balance and stability. I prefer to perform two to three core exercises with each of my workouts, usually right after my warm-up, as it helps prepare me for the bulk of my exercise routine.

If you're new to exercise, perform core exercises at the end of your workout until you gain enough strength in your abs and back to prevent early workout fatigue in these muscles.

Exhausting your core muscles, while appropriate for the more advanced exerciser, could prevent you from maintaining correct form on your other exercises, since your core muscles are critical for maintaining good posture. This could result in a serious injury, so take it slow in the beginning with core training.

Combined stretching and resistance training is an excellent way to kill two birds with one stone. A really good example is the practice of yoga. In yoga, you stretch your muscles but also hold sustained and demanding poses in such a way that your entire body is strengthened. Personally, I love yoga and bring it into my workout routine once or twice a week.

The human body is highly adaptive when it comes to exercise. If you do the same routine every time you work out, your body and mind will go on autopilot and you'll see fewer results. If you're going to take the time to work out, why waste your time? Do it right and mix it up!

MAXIMUM HEART RATE

Your heart carries oxygen-filled blood from your lungs and pumps it throughout your system. It then carries blood filled with carbon dioxide (an odorless gas) from your body's extremities to your lungs where the carbon dioxide is released as you exhale.

Your diet and exercise program directly affect the health of your heart. Your heart is a muscle so, just like any other muscle, it benefits from regular workouts.

People who participate in both anaerobic and aerobic exercise typically have resting heart rates of around 60 beats per minute. A person who doesn't exercise will have a heart rate of around 80 beats per minute or higher, depending on other health choices such as whether they smoke and how well they eat. A low resting heart rate is an important measure of good health.

The health of your heart also depends on its size and how well it is supplied with blood vessels. An athlete's heart is strong and healthy. It's relatively large and highly efficient at pumping more blood with each contraction (thus its lower resting rate). It takes less effort for an athlete's heart to pump blood than that of a non-athlete; in other words, a fitter heart is more efficient. So how do you get a strong and healthy heart? By eating right and exercising, of course.

To this end, it's important to know your maximum heart rate (MHR) so you can avoid either underperforming or overdoing it as you exercise. Your MHR is the highest rate at which your heart is able to beat in one minute. To calculate what your maximum heart rate is, subtract your age from the number 220. For example, if you're 30 years old your maximum heart rate is 190 beats per minute. This method produces a good estimation of your MHR; there are more complex ways to get a more accurate number, but for the purposes of this program the preceding formula is more than sufficient.

Exercise heart rates are usually categorized into different

"zones" of effectiveness, which you will often see printed on cardio equipment or posters at your gym. These typically include:

- **Fitness zone:** This is considered the fat-burning zone. Here, your heart rate count-per-minute while exercising is around 60 to 70 percent of your MHR. Try to reach this level of intensity, at a minimum, while performing cardiovascular training or exercise. This will help you to burn your fat stores more efficiently. (Note that the term "fat-burning zone" is frequently misunderstood. The so-called fat-burning zone is not the only heart rate range where fat burning will occur. Remember, if you're exercising whatsoever, you're burning fat. It's just at varying rates.)

- **Aerobic zone:** In this endurance-training zone your exercise heart rate is around 70 to 80 percent of your MHR. This is the perfect zone for those seeking to improve their cardiovascular and respiratory fitness. This zone also strengthens your heart and allows it to function better.

- **Anaerobic zone:** Also known as the performance-training zone, working in this zone will improve your cardio-respiratory system and help you fight fatigue. In this high-intensity zone your exercise heart rate reaches 80 to 90 percent of your MHR, allowing you to burn even more food-derived energy (i.e., calories).

- **Red line:** In this zone your body is putting forth its maximum effort as you work at 90 to 100 percent of your MHR. Unless you've been exercising for years and currently have a high fitness level, you should not be in this zone. Check with your doctor before pushing your body to this level.

If you're new to exercise, I highly recommend that you purchase a heart rate monitor so you can tell exactly which zone you're in. You can purchase a good monitor for $30 to $60 at most athletic stores. There are different styles of heart rate monitors, each designed for different types of athletic event. The most common model resembles a watch that's worn on your wrist, although other models can be worn around your waist or upper arm.

If you belong to a gym, you can also use the built-in monitors on the cardio machines. Most modern cardiovascular exercise equipment has a heart rate monitor built into its handle. If you're unsure how to use it, or have a question, ask a gym employee to help you.

RESISTANCE TRAINING: BULKING UP VERSUS TONING UP

Resistance training is sometimes referred to as strength training or weight training. This type of exercise increases your muscular strength with weights (resistance) such as dumbbells, barbells, resistance bands or your own body weight.

Resistance training can increase muscle strength and bone density, as well as produce denser, stronger muscles. This is not to knock aerobic exercise; that's also very important. However, many people underestimate the value of incorporating resistance training into their workouts, and I don't want you to make the same mistake. The bottom line is that you will get the best results when you combine both aerobic and resistance training for a synergistic training effect.

Many people mistakenly think that only bodybuilders should lift heavy weights. Time and time again, new gym-goers say, "I don't want to lift weights or do resistance training because it will make me look bulky." Women especially have this fear, since many of them want to have a more streamlined athletic look.

However, the belief that lifting weights automatically leads to bulky muscles is a complete myth, particularly in the case of women. Creating the muscular look of a bodybuilder takes years and years of intense physical training, a great deal of dedication, protein and supplements, and a deep understanding of human biochemistry. Nobody looks like that without years of extremely intense, multi-hour, daily workouts. Working out with weights three to four times per week will **not** turn you into a hulking green superhero running around in shredded pants, I promise you!

You will, however, look slimmer and more toned and feel much stronger and more energetic. Resistance training is an essential part of efficient weight loss and the maintenance of a balanced, healthy body.

EXERCISE SEQUENCING

There are several theories as to the optimal combination and sequence of targeted resistance exercises. However, we'll leave that discussion to the realms of bodybuilders and elite athletes. To get you going on a basic and healthy routine, I have provided you with some starter workouts that are safe, achievable and effective.

Muscle groups are generally broken up by fitness professionals into the groups outlined below. Thus we will target the following muscles, one at a time:

- Biceps

- Triceps

- Legs, including your calves

- Back

- Shoulders

- Chest

- Abdominals (abs)

A quick note: The primary reasons to warm up and stretch at the beginning of each workout are to prevent injury and prepare the muscles for physical activity. Warming up and stretching properly boost blood circulation and elongate muscles in preparation for your activity.

New exercisers often jump right in and start working out without first warming up or stretching because they mistakenly feel these preparatory steps are unnecessary. Then once their main, higher-intensity activity is complete, they typically don't cool down. However, I urge you not to make these novice mistakes! Whether it's a low-impact or intense workout you're doing, it's important to warm up, cool down and stretch.

An example of a good warm-up, stretch and cool-down routine is as follows: Warm up with some cardio, and then perform some light stretching before beginning your resistance training. I recommend light stretching to prepare the joints and muscle for resistance training. In the past, exercise professionals have recommended longer, static stretching before resistance training. However, I've found this can actually overstretch muscles and loosen joint connective tissue, thus weakening the stability of joints, which can possibly lead to injury. Performing your cardio first like this is a great way to warm up *and* get some aerobic training in at the same time

After you've completed your resistance training, perform five to ten minutes of light cardio (as a cool-down) and then do another round of light stretching. This type of routine helps avoid injuries.

A special note on abs: I recommend including abdominal exercises in your workout routine a minimum of two to three times per week. Then, over time as you build up strength, try to include abdominals in every workout. But remember, you cannot "spot-reduce" fat from your stomach area by doing abdominal exercises. Only a proper diet, combined with exercise, can give you a six-pack!

Below are two sample exercise routines. The first one is recommended for those of you just starting out. The second one is for those already at a more advanced fitness level, or who are stuck on a pound-loss plateau.

Something is Always Better Than Nothing

Now to the nuts and bolts of your personal exercise plan. While the old school recommended 30 minutes of exercise, three times a week, is enough to create minimal health benefits, it typically isn't enough for weight loss or real fitness results. You need to perform at least four to five hours of exercise per week to truly see benefits in your life.

However, if you can't find at least four hours to spare, you can still do something. Start with what you *can* do, no matter what. When it comes to doing nothing versus doing at least something, remember that something is always the right choice.

A special note on the term "rest days": You will see that the recommended exercise routines that follow include days reserved for rest. One rest day, in workout terms, doesn't involve sitting still and doing nothing. Rather, it means that you shouldn't do any resistance training, or any challenging cardio such as running or sprinting, on that day.

You can, however, still do light, low-intensity movement on a rest day. I recommend going for a short bike ride or a walk, as long as this is a low-intensity activity for you. Try to do so after dinner if possible, to help relieve the stress of the day and assist with digestion. Once your body becomes more adapted to exercise, you can take on more challenging cardiovascular activities on your rest days, but keep it basic and easy for now.

Rest days are essential to your long-term improvements in strength. It's during the rests between your workouts that your body can get to the important business of repairing and strengthening muscles and replenishing essential energy stores. It's the proper balance of the right intensity of work (exercise) followed by restful activities that will give you the best results.

Finally, if you're feeling really run-down or are coming down with a cold, you should take a break and get some rest. Your body will thank you and be revived for your next exercise session.

WORKOUT #1: TRUE BEGINNERS

The text below is not intended to give you an entire workout routine, but more of a guideline on what a beginner workout routine should look like.

A quick note: A *repetition (rep)* is one complete movement of an exercise, such as a single bicep curl. A *set* is the total number of repetitions you perform for that exercise.

Day 1

Biceps, back, triceps and calves. Two to three sets of each, 10 to 12 reps per set, 30 to 45 seconds of rest between each set. 15 to 30 minutes of cardio.

A note on cardio: If you haven't exercised in years, or have never participated in a workout program, start with a maximum of 10 to 15 minutes of cardio per workout day.

Day 2
Rest day

Day 3
Chest, shoulders, legs and abs. Two to three sets of each, 10 to 12 reps, 30 to 45 seconds of rest between each set. 15 to 30 minutes of cardio (or 10 to 15 for true beginners).

Day 4
Rest day

Day 5
Biceps, back, triceps and calves. Two to three sets of each, 10 to 12 reps, 30 to 45 seconds of rest between each set. 15 to 30 minutes of cardio (or 10 to 15 for true beginners).

Day 6
Rest day

Day 7
Chest, shoulders, legs and abs. Two to three sets of each, 10 to 12 reps, 30 to 45 seconds of rest between each set. 15 to 30 minutes of cardio (or 10 to 15 for true beginners).

WORKOUT #2: A MORE ADVANCED ROUTINE

Day 1
Biceps, back and calves. Two to three sets of each, 8 to 10 reps, 15 to 30 seconds of rest between each set. 20 to 35 minutes of cardio, such as speed walking, running, bike riding, or using other cardio equipment if you belong to a gym.

Day 2
Chest, triceps and abs. Two to three sets of each, 8 to 10 reps, 15 to 30 seconds of rest between each set. 20 to 35 minutes of cardio.

Day 3

Rest day

Day 4

Legs, shoulders and calves. Two to three sets of each, 8 to 10 reps, 15 to 30 seconds of rest between each set. 20 to 35 minutes of cardio.

Day 5

Biceps, back and calves. Two to three sets of each, 8 to 10 reps, 15 to 30 seconds of rest between each set. 20 to 35 minutes of cardio.

Day 6

Chest, triceps and abs. Two to three sets of each, 8 to 10 reps, 15 to 30 seconds of rest between each set. 20 to 35 minutes of cardio.

Day 7

Rest day

For those of you who have limited space, I recommend you purchase a jump rope, as they're great for instant cardio and can be taken anywhere.

For now, don't be intimidated when starting a new exercise program. It's normal to feel a little uneasy about something new that you may not completely understand. I know I was lost the first time I ever joined a gym, although I realized there was no shortcut to optimal fitness. Be patient as you gain more knowledge and experience, and working out will become easier over time.

To help you a little more, I've provided a list of different types of activities and how many calories each one burns. Wait, Gary, didn't you say I don't need to count calories earlier? Yes, this is just to give you an idea of the different amounts of energy expended on whatever exercises you decide to do.

The Caloric Expenditure of Common Activities

Activity (1 hour)	Calories burned, 130 lb. person	Calories burned, 155 lb. person	Calories burned, 190 lb. person
Aerobics, general	354	422	518
Backpacking, general	413	493	604
Basketball, game	472	563	690
Bicycling, moderate effort	472	563	690
Bicycling, BMX or mountain	502	598	733
Calisthenics, home, light/moderate	266	317	388
Canoeing, rowing, moderate effort	413	493	604
Circuit training, general	472	563	690
Dancing, general	266	317	388
Football, touch, flag, general	472	563	690
Golf, general	236	281	345
Jogging, general	413	493	604
Judo, karate, kickboxing, taekwondo	590	704	863
Racquetball, casual	413	493	604
Rock climbing, ascending rock	649	774	949
Rope jumping, moderate	590	704	863
Running, general	472	563	690
Running, up stairs	885	1056	1294
Skateboarding	295	352	431
Skating, ice, general	413	493	604
Skiing, cross-country, moderate	472	563	690
Skiing, snow, general	413	493	604
Skiing, water	354	422	518
Snorkeling	295	352	431
Soccer, moderate	413	493	604
Stretching, hatha yoga	236	281	345
Surfing, bodyboarding	177	211	259

Swimming laps, freestyle, moderate	472	563	690
Tennis, general	413	493	604
Volleyball, beach	472	563	690
Walking, running, playing, with children	236	281	345
Water aerobics, water calisthenics	236	281	345
Weightlifting, light or moderate	177	211	259
Whitewater rafting, kayaking, canoeing	295	352	431

Source: International Sports Science Association, Nutrition: The Complete Guide (Carpinteria: International Sports Science Association, 2009).

Beyond the Basics

In my experience in the fitness industry, I've found that the simple workouts previously discussed are the easiest for people to follow, understand and stick with. However, there are many different types of exercise routines out there.

As you advance in your exercise knowledge and skill level, you'll begin to experiment with different amounts of reps, sets, training schedules, and incorporating different exercise routines. Don't be afraid to change the combination of body parts you exercise after you master the above examples. Mix it up to keep your body challenged. You don't have to perform chest exercises with triceps every time, for example; you can combine your chest workout with biceps, your back or any other body part.

I continuously mix up my body part combinations to keep my workouts fresh and exciting. Also, remember that the more athletic styles of yoga and interval training are types of resistance training as well, so don't be afraid to mix in other strength-based exercises that you like.

SOME EXERCISE AND TRAINING TIPS

Social Circles and Joining a Gym

Another obstacle you'll face is your social circles. Studies have repeatedly shown that people's life accomplishments directly correlate to the quality of the company they keep most of the time. This is especially true when it comes to dietary habits and exercise.

But therein lies the solution: A combination of good nutrition, a well-devised exercise program and a strong social support network is a winning combination for transforming your body and mind.

You're more likely to stick with this program and complete it if you're surrounded by people who are trying to accomplish or maintain similar health goals. When an individual is serious about getting healthy and the people near and dear are not supportive, that person almost always fails to improve their fitness and well-being.

Now, this is not about severing relationships with family and friends who are unconcerned with health or nutrition. Simply, if you find yourself alone in your goals amongst family and friends, you'll need to find an alternative social group who will be supportive and help keep you motivated. One good way to achieve this is to encourage your family and friends to do the program with you!

If your current social network is a major obstacle, I highly recommend you join a gym. Why? People at the gym are probably there for the same reason you are: to get in shape. Not only will you be surrounded by like-minded folks, but you might also meet new friends and professionals who can assist you in your health and nutrition goals.

If you do decide to join a gym, do your homework and find the right gym for you. It should have a positive environment that's supportive of the goals you're trying to accomplish. There's no magic formula for finding the right facility. You just have to physically go to each gym in your area and try them out to see which one will best suit your needs.

Most gyms are listed on the Internet and can be searched with key words like "gyms" or "health clubs." Don't rule out smaller, private gyms. They may, however, be harder to find than the locations of a major chain and may only have one facility.

Narrow it down to two or three gyms and try them out for a couple of weeks before you decide which one you want to join. Each gym will have its own social culture and personality, so it's important that you find one that suits you. If you can find a family member or friend to join with you, gyms often offer discounts for a friend or family member package. Best of all, your exercise time can lead to life-long friendships with like-minded people. If you have the financial resources to join a gym, I definitely recommend you do so.

Avoiding Workout Distractions

When working out, you'll get better results if you maintain a total focus on exercise, rather than on the rest of the world.

To this end, my biggest pet peeve when it comes to working out is the use of cell phones and smart phones in the gym. Unless you're someone whose profession requires people to contact you in emergency situations, your cell phone should not be with you as you work out. Besides being bad gym etiquette, your cell phone detracts from your ability to get a good workout, which is the whole reason you're there in the first place.

It drives me absolutely nuts when I see people chatting on their cell phone or checking their social media status when they should be focused on getting a good sweat. How are you going to concentrate on your exercise technique with a cell phone in your hand or against your ear the entire time? You're not—you're just wasting your time! (Of course, if you're exercising outdoors you should always carry a cell phone for emergency purposes. *Note:* social media updates are not an emergency!)

This principle of staying focused on the workout at hand not only applies to the use of cell phones, but also to avoiding the distractions of magazines, newspapers or anything else that could shift your focus away from your real goal of getting fit. Of course I'm not an exercise sadist; I understand that your music is probably on your phone. But that's not what I'm talking about.

Use your workouts as a way of tuning out the world for a while and focusing on you. You'll notice working out is the best stress reliever around. Take advantage of some precious you-time by eliminating everyday distractions and you'll get so much more out of your time at the gym.

HIRING A PERSONAL TRAINER

If you think the exercise portion of this program may be difficult to follow, or if you want an extra push, consider hiring a personal trainer (PT). Hiring a trainer is a great idea if your finances allow. Here are some basic guidelines for getting the right help.

1. The most important trait of a good PT is that he or she practices what they preach. I've seen far too many trainers over the years in terrible physical shape. If you can't maintain and follow the principles you're attempting to teach, odds are that you're not passionate about what you do. Would you want someone managing your finances that is bankrupt and doesn't pay his or her own bills? I hope not!

2. Make sure the PT has a personality that works well with yours. If you feel uncomfortable during your training sessions, it will be difficult for you to get the results you want. It will be also hard to remain motivated, which could be detrimental to your goals. If this happens, just ask to work with a different trainer. Gyms understand that this happens from time to time and are usually very accommodating.

3. Beware of the trainer who is pushing the latest physical workout fad and is not open to any other exercise ideas. This reluctance is probably an indicator that he or she doesn't understand other concepts in exercise science and can only work from one workout template.

CrossFit training has been around for a while now, and it consists of a strength and conditioning program that combines powerlifting, sprinting, gymnastics, rowing and medicine ball training. Don't get me wrong—this can be a great exercise method for an athlete or someone competing in organized sports. However, giving this type of program to every enthusiast, regardless of his or her level of experience or fitness, is unproductive and potentially harmful.

If CrossFit is something you're interested in, make sure you're physically ready for such a challenge and you have a Box (Cross-Fit gym) referred to you by someone who belongs to that one. CrossFit Boxes can be drastically different in their approach and experience in exercise.

I witnessed a PT put a 60-year-old, overweight female through this type of program, and I was cringing the entire time. How will an aggressive exercise program benefit someone in that type of physical condition? She'll probably end up burned out at best, and injured at worst.

If your trainer pushes you beyond reasonable limits of safety, tell them you're not interested in running a faster 40-yard dash or in completing a Marine-worthy obstacle course. Make sure the program your PT designs is tailored to *your* goals, not theirs.

Including Exercise in Your Family Plans When You Can

One of the most common exercise excuses is lack of time, but consider that the average American watches over four hours of television per day. In this case, not having enough time is an excuse that just doesn't resonate with me. Most of us spend over one day per week watching television. So I'm sure you can find three to four hours out of that time to do something more productive—like exercise!

But let's suppose you're super busy with work and family commitments and don't even have extra time to turn on the TV. If you're like me and have very little time to spare, try this: Rather than trying to *find* time to exercise, try to *fit* exercise into your existing family and work routines. Here are some exercise suggestions for super busy people with family and work commitments:

- Try to take a walk every night after dinner, and include your partner, pets and/or kids in the activity. Not only does this after-dinner stroll help with digestion, it can be great bonding time for a family. Don't let a cold or rainy climate stop you—just invest in the right kinds of outdoor clothes and enjoy moving in the fresh air.

- Instead of zoning out on movies or video games, plan family activities around kid-friendly exercise such as bike rides, playing in the park, or just playing physically active games in your yard. You don't have to be in a gym to get your heart pumping, and you'll be teaching your kids the value of healthy movement.

- On your lunch break, hit the gym or go for a run or a jog. If you're short on time and don't have access to a shower, at least go for a short walk outside in your office clothes. Remember, something is always better than nothing, and every step counts!

- Plan to exercise during your children's naps or after they go to bed. Just let the dirty dishes and laundry pile up from time to time and get moving. Remember, your health is more important than a spotless house!

- Run, walk or ride your bike to and from work, if possible. You'll lose weight and save a lot of gas money in the process. Another trick if your work is a long way from your home is to park a reasonable distance from your office, then walk, jog, run or ride your bike the remainder of the way.

It's important that you plan a realistic exercise schedule that's in harmony with your everyday activities and responsibilities. If you don't, it's easy to miss a couple of days and then fall into old sedentary habits. Once you've established your routine it becomes easier and easier to keep going, since movement will then be an integral part of your and your family's daily activities.

Family exercise time is not the only way to be a role model to your children. It's just as important that they learn healthy eating habits from you as well. After all, if they don't find out about proper nutrition from you, how will your kids learn to live energetic and healthy lives?

Of course, we all have bad days when plans go awry. However, I've almost always been able to squeeze in a little exercise every day, no matter what, even if it's just a short walk. I truly believe one of the best gifts you can give your kids and loved ones is to be an exercise role model and demonstrate the value of healthy movement. It just takes a bit of time management and dedication to get there.

Finding Balance Between Workouts and Work

I know from personal experience that it can be very hard to fit it all in. Nevertheless, it's so worth it.

For example, during my career in the federal government, exercising was very important to me for relief from my day-to-day stress. Most of the time while traveling out of town for work, I could find a gym nearby. However, even when I didn't have access to a full fitness center, I did what I could, taking 30-minute runs, doing some sit-ups and push-ups, or using exercise bands. I always felt better after completing my midday workout, since it helped release the tension I had built up throughout the day.

Here's my million-dollar tip to stay on track with no excuses: The way I made sure that I could pretty much work out anytime, anywhere, was to have what I called my "workout survival kit." This was simply a set of workout clothes, a pair of running shoes, a jump rope and a set of resistance bands. I kept this in the trunk of my work car in a gym bag that was separate from my daily workout change of clothes. So, say if I forgot my workout clothes that day, I had my workout survival kit ready to go. Not only that, but if I was really busy doing surveillance or working in a neighboring city, I had my workout survival kit to get in a quick workout at a park or outdoor recreational area.

Doing Things You Enjoy

The best way to make sure you will stick with any exercise program is to do things you enjoy. No, that doesn't mean curling cheeseburgers and beers! What I mean is incorporating types of exercise that you look forward to doing. For me, I love road biking, mountain biking, hiking/walking with my dog, and lifting weights. So guess what I do? Yep, I incorporate all the activities that I enjoy into my exercise routine.

Making it Happen

You need to be adaptable! Your workout program or routine should never suffer because of your schedule. Being very busy is why a lot of people get off track or stop exercising altogether. Being busy will always be a reality in our lives; we need to plan around this, not succumb to the phenomenon.

Remember, if you miss a workout the world won't end. Just get back on track right away and do your missed workout on the next day. From time to time I have missed several workouts in a row due to my work schedule. But I didn't just throw in the towel. I picked up where I left off when I had the time again.

Missing a couple of days here and there is not going to make you gain weight or get completely out of shape. It's what you do over the long term that really counts!

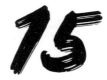

Should I Take Supplements in Order to Be Healthy?

The cornerstone of your ultimate success lies in a natural, whole-foods diet and consistent workout habits. There is absolutely no magic supplement or miracle powdered drink that will make up for a junk food diet or a total lack of exercise; period. However, I believe high-quality supplements, vitamins and protein powders can be powerful and positive complements to a solid overall health program. I've been taking supplements in one form or another for over three decades. Bottom line: Some are good, some are junk.

The discussion of what has gone wrong in our food supply is, slowly but surely, bubbling up to the surface of our national health care conversation. Quality organic food is becoming more readily available, and more people are gradually becoming aware that the modern, conventional way of eating is making us fatter ...and killing us.

In a perfect world, we'd all eat a diet based upon freshly-picked, locally-grown organic vegetables, fruits, legumes and nuts, complemented by the meat, eggs and dairy products of organically and humanely raised animals. I talk about these ideas a lot because the preceding sentence, coupled with exercise, really represents the proverbial holy grail of health.

However, we don't live in an ideal world. Not all of us have access to (or the funds for) the quality of foods we should be eating—the quality that your great-grandparents, who didn't have access to processed junk, most likely ate. Making matters worse, few of us have much extra time to prepare homemade meals and snacks each and every day.

Moreover, if you eat poorly, it's likely that you're deficient in key vitamins and minerals. In addition, studies show that today's soils produce foods with about 30 percent fewer nutrients than those of a century ago. This is due to soil degradation (a natural or human-caused reduction in soil quality) and to the use of modern pesticides and chemicals. So even if you are eating a healthy diet, it's still possible that your nutrient intake is insufficient. For this reason, I recommend taking a well-rounded multivitamin every day.

So how do you split the difference between what's *ideal* and what's *real*? In an imperfect situation, for those times that our best efforts to eat what we know is ideal fall short, there are practical, real-world strategies you can use to work around the lack of time we all experience and to mitigate the shortcomings of our failing food supply.

A big part of these strategies is the use of *nutritional supplements* (also known as a *dietary* or *food supplements*). These are products that aim to make up for, or supplement, certain nutrients in your diet, such as protein, fatty acids or vitamins. Nutritional supplements may be botanicals (natural herbs), vitamins, minerals, amino acids, enzymes or fatty acids, to name a few examples.

They're often sold as pills (such as vitamins), powders (like protein powders), bars (as in protein or energy bars), or in a drinkable liquid form.

My Tried-and-True Supplement List that I Think Everyone Can Benefit From

What dietary supplements can almost everyone benefit from? Here's my list of top choices to consider for your optimal health goals:

- Multivitamin

- Vitamin D3 (75 percent of Americans are found to be deficient)

- Fish oil (omega 3)

- Green food supplements (greens)

- Probiotics

- Turmeric (a potent cancer-fighting and anti-inflammatory spice)

I also encourage you to consider occasionally using a high-quality protein powder to complement your dietary efforts, and as a healthier alternative to eating fast food when you're on the run.

In the next section, I'll tell you what to look for when complementing your whole-foods meals with vitamins, protein powders and other dietary supplements.

WHAT SHOULD YOU SHOULD LOOK FOR WHEN PURCHASING SUPPLEMENTS?

This isn't everything to consider, but everything here is easy to determine and important when it comes to quality. Look for as many of these criteria as possible:

- Made in the U.S.A.

- Organic, when possible

- Non-GMO

- Gluten-free

- No added sugars or artificial sweeteners

- Made from natural, whole food sources (not chemicals)

- Product contact information clearly displayed on the supplement label and manufacturer's website

How to Avoid Poor Quality Supplements

- Avoid products endorsed by a famous actor, singer or model. Choose quality, not celebrity.

- Don't buy cheap supplements. It takes money to make a safe, effective health product. It's no bargain if a cheaply made supplement costs you your well-being.

- Avoid over-the-top, miracle weight-loss claims. If it sounds too good to be true, it is.

- Research the manufacturer and look for a U.S.-based address and phone number. Always purchase supplements manufactured in the U.S, or that have strong U.S ties.

This is not a perfect way to avoid counterfeit and cheap supplements, but it's far better than buying supplements that are produced outside of the U.S.

- If you regularly purchase a supplement and then find it somewhere else for a much lower price, beware. This is usually a telltale sign that the cheap product is a counterfeit or a repackaged expired product.

WHY YOU SHOULD BE CAREFUL WHEN PURCHASING SUPPLEMENTS ON AMAZON OR EBAY

When I first published an article, years ago, on my experience dealing with counterfeit supplements as a special agent for the U.S. Food and Drug Administration, I was surprised by the response, as the article was shared well over 100,000 times. I mainly focused on purchasing supplements on Amazon, but included eBay as well. At the time, Amazon was fairly new at listing food or supplement products for sale. So, needless to say, it was a counterfeiter's—and dirty supplement seller's—paradise.

A lot has changed since then, so I felt it was important to include an updated summary of that article in this book, because now Amazon pretty much sells everything, including a lot of food products and supplements.

Things have gotten somewhat better, but that doesn't mean everything is fine and it's OK to buy any supplement you can find on Amazon. There are still things to be cautious about anytime you're buying supplements online. And, in my opinion, even though eBay is changing its business model, I would still not buy supplements or food products there. After all I've seen and learned, it just seems like a really bad idea to me.

I've been behind the curtain of the supplement industry—way

behind—so what I say is not based on some far-fetched conspiracy theory. I was there and witnessed it firsthand. So I want to share some insider information on how the dark side of the supplement industry works.

There are three main ways that supplements end up on the market at unbelievably cheap prices:

1. They are counterfeit and probably dangerous.

2. They are useless, expired products that have been repackaged as new.

3. They are stolen products released on the black market without any quality control.

Here's how each scenario plays out:

Counterfeit Products

One of the easiest ways to make a dishonest buck in the supplement world is to create a pill that mirrors a name-brand health supplement. Create look-alike packaging and you can sell your worthless pill on the Internet for a "discounted" price—and a counterfeit operation is born!

People would be appalled if they knew how prevalent counterfeit dietary supplements truly are. Sadly, fake vitamins and "health" capsules have made their way into the general consumer market.

These dangerous pills masquerade as the real thing on the shelves of the name-brand department stores that virtually every family in America patronizes—and they certainly are available on the Internet.

Here's the bottom line: If an above-board supplement or pharmaceutical drug is popular, you can bet someone, primarily in China or India, is counterfeiting it. I'm not saying this as some off-the-wall scare tactic. I was there and this was my job.

Even worse? Fake pills virtually never have the correct amount of the active ingredient they are supposed to contain.

During my FDA tenure, we ran lab tests on all kinds of look-alike pills and capsules. Some cheap/counterfeit supplements had ten times or more the amount of medicinal ingredients that were indicated on the label. Worse, some had none, and others simply contained large amounts of sawdust!

Criminals are not moral, but they're often smart. They not only counterfeit health supplements, but also all of the paperwork that goes along with them. They have numerous distribution shell companies set up all over the world, so it's almost impossible to figure out the paperwork trail and the actual origins of these dangerous pills. (Trust me, I've been paid to untangle this kind of web many times.)

The real-world result is that there are virtually no legal consequences to selling fake pills, capsules or vitamins, and the criminals know it.

How prevalent are fake supplements? The IACC (International Anti-Counterfeiting Coalition) estimates that brand-holders (the legitimate companies behind name-brand, non-counterfeit products) lose approximately $600 billion of revenue annually because of counterfeiting.

Michael Danel, the secretary general of the World Customs Organization, has said that if terrorism didn't exist, counterfeiting would be the most significant criminal act of the early twenty-first century.

That's why it's so important to buy directly from a legitimate manufacturer or from a trusted health practitioner whenever you can. Bottom line: If it seems fake, it probably is. And if it's really cheap, it's almost certainly a counterfeit.

Expired Products

Another way to make a dishonest living is to purchase a genuine product that's expired, for pennies on the dollar. Change the date on the package label and voila: You have a cheap "new" product ready to be brought back to market.

Legitimate supplement companies often have fire sales when they have products that are about to expire. The counterfeiters love this, as it fits right into their business model. They can purchase these legitimate products and package them with counterfeit products and no one is the wiser.

I've seen this done in a couple of ways: The criminals might simply replace the label with a new label and a fictitious expiration date. Or, if they received the expired product in raw form (not in the bottle), they will sometimes mix it with counterfeit tablets or capsules.

Bottom line: If criminals can make a couple of bucks on something, they will. It all boils down to money. And by purchasing expired, legitimate products, they can have "genuine" products on hand if something goes wrong and someone complains.

Once again, it's the consumer who pays the price.

Stolen Products Resold by Criminal Enterprises

This scheme is pretty straightforward: Criminals simply break into the warehouse of an above-board supplement company, or take a big rig truck transporting nutritional products by force. They then distribute the products to other criminal fencing enterprises, and the supplements end up on the Internet at a super cheap price.

Alternatively, employees of a genuine supplement company might steal products while at work and then sell them on the black market to criminals.

You may think, well in this case it's a genuine supplement, so why should I care? Here's why: Criminals don't just work with stolen products, but with expired and counterfeit products as well. They all get mixed together.

So you, as the consumer, will never know which variation of the product you're getting. You may get lucky one time; another time you may not be so lucky. Is it really worth your health to save a couple of bucks? Absolutely not!

What My FDA Experience Taught Me

The sad truth is that fake-pill-pushing criminals often operate in countries at a distance far further than Uncle Sam's laws can reach. It's easy to sell counterfeit supplements at reputable online venues such as Amazon and eBay. But for the consumer, it's a disaster.

Here's what a decade of forensic investigation really taught me: Your instincts are usually right. If you can't easily trace the origins of some "miracle" pills, or are given the runaround by a supplement sales rep when you ask complex questions about ingredients or packaging, your gut will tell you what's up. Go with your gut.

Whomever you choose to purchase supplements from, please research their products meticulously first. The supplement descriptions on *The Simple Life* website offer a template of what to look for in each product category. Only use the best quality items that meet these criteria.

Take it from a guy who has worked way behind the curtain and seen the proverbial puppet strings: You don't want to mess around when it comes to taking any kind of dietary supplement; period. Insist on the best—your health depends on it.

Is There a Place Where I Can Purchase Safe and Healthy Supplements?

I've been selling my own line of supplements for several years now. I originally started doing this when I realized my clients were going out and buying all kinds of junk supplements and derailing all the hard work we had been putting into their health programs. So I did what made sense—I created my own high-quality line that included all the supplements I had been taking for years... and that actually work!

For those who are interested in the supplements I recommended earlier in this chapter, you can find them in a handy-dandy all-in-one package at **www.thesimplelifenow.com**.

None of my supplements are sold anywhere except for on my website, so if you see them somewhere else they are 100% fake; period. Sure, I lose money with this business model, but I know for sure my supplements come from one place... me!

16

Intermittent Fasting and the Ketogenic State

I constantly get asked about fasting, especially intermittent fasting, usually by people looking to shortcut the initial stages of acquiring better health or trying to lose weight quickly. Fasting and intermittent fasting are often used by trendy personal trainers, or supposed health experts, as a quick-fix technique, without knowing the theory and premise behind these strategies. There's a physiological reason why fasting works and can be a natural progression as you gain more experience at bettering your health. That is, if it's done correctly.

This topic is usually very confusing, especially for those just starting a weight-loss or exercise program. That's why I never recommend that beginners incorporate or start an intermittent—or any—fasting program. That being said, I do think such a program can have many benefits for those who have mastered the basic principles of *The Simple Life Healthy Lifestyle Plan*.

I have personally experimented with fasting over the last several years and consistently use intermittent fasting as a way to stay in fat-burning mode. I don't do it every single day, but I do it a majority of the time, depending on my physical exercise exertion and how I feel.

What I'm about to cover will be a departure from the usual information concerning proper nutrition. For those of you unfamiliar with this concept of fasting, I only ask that you keep an open mind, as there is no specific program that works for everyone. When it comes to health and wellness, this is simply another tool to add to your knowledge base.

WHAT IS INTERMITTENT FASTING?

So what is *intermittent fasting*? It's often called *periodic fasting*, and both terms are interchangeable as they basically refer to the same concept: periods of not consuming any foods (usually only consuming water, black coffee or unsweetened tea), followed by eating fewer meals than usual, during a certain time frame. This is not to be confused with actual fasting, which is when you don't consume any food for 24 to 36 hours (or longer).

There are many theories on how to schedule eating during intermittent fasting, but we'll stick to the most basic and widely used schedule of 16–8. 16–8 basically means 16 hours of fasting, followed by eating all your meals in an 8-hour window. Usually people who follow this type of schedule eat their last meal at anywhere from 5 p.m. to 8 p.m., then fast until late morning (usually between 9 a.m. and 12 p.m.) or until roughly 16 hours of fasting is completed. Everyone's schedule is different, though, so you have to figure out what works for you.

How Does It Work?

The basic premise is that intermittent fasting kickstarts your metabolism by keeping your body in a fat-burning mode (keto-genic state) for longer periods of time. By not eating for 16 hours, your body will burn through its glucose stores and will use available glycogen (when needed), along with stored fat, as the body's main sources of energy. Of course, this only works if you're eating a healthy diet. If you're eating a diet high in sugar and processed white flour or carbohydrates, you'll never obtain your health and weight-loss goals, no matter what type of fasting or exercise program you follow. If you have constant elevated blood sugar, thus elevated insulin levels, you'll store more and more body fat over time.

In 2011, researchers at the Intermountain Medical Center Heart Institute demonstrated that routine periodic fasting burns body fat and is good for your health:

> *"Fasting causes hunger or stress. In response, the body releases more cholesterol, allowing it to utilize fat as a source of fuel instead of glucose. This decreases the number of fat cells in the body," says Dr. Horne. "This is important because the fewer fat cells a body has, the less likely it will experience insulin resistance or diabetes."*

In order to get the full benefits, people should combine inter-mittent fasting with a solid exercise program. Upon waking, instead of eating breakfast, you go to the gym or incorporate some type of exercise prior to your first meal of the day, which is technically lunch. By exercising near the end of your 16-hour fast, you kick your body into fat-burning overdrive, as you no longer are using readily available blood glucose as fuel.

The concept is this: When you eat consistently throughout the day, you're constantly dumping glucose into your bloodstream, never allowing it to drop low enough for your body to go after your stored body fat as an energy source.

In order to avoid going into a prolonged catabolic state, which is breaking down muscle for fuel, I do recommend you consume a recovery meal within 1.5 to 2 hours after you exercise, especially if you're trying to build muscle. If you're a competitive athlete, I recommend consuming something within 30 to 60 minutes after you train or exercise. This can get a little tricky if you're exercising first thing in the morning, so you'll need to plan your fasting hours accordingly by properly timing your last meal of the day.

When I know I'll be on the run after my workout, or not able to eat within the 1.5- to 2-hour window, I usually carry a protein shake in my gym bag. My protein shake will typically consist of coconut milk, almond butter, some berries and protein powder. This recovery meal contains a quick-digesting protein, healthy fats, carbohydrates and fiber. These vital macronutrients give my body what it requires to maintain and repair muscle and restore energy levels.

If you feel you have low energy before your workout, I recommend eating a small snack or drinking some black coffee, or green tea with a teaspoon of coconut oil; this will ensure you have enough energy for a good workout. It's essential that you eat something before exercising if you feel lightheaded; even I've experienced this from time to time, and I have years of fasting experience.

CAN INTERMITTENT FASTING SLOW THE AGING PROCESS?

In the last several years, more research has been done on 24-hour and intermittent fasting and how it relates to stomach fat loss, anti-aging, increased HDL levels (good cholesterol), reduced blood pressure, reduced blood sugar and improved insulin sensitivity.

When you incorporate fasting into your health and wellness program, you need to realize you are putting your body into a catabolic state, which means your body is feeding off its tissues to maintain energy and life-supporting needs. Research shows that when you combine fasting with exercise, your body is forced to break down its tissues, and it always prefers to sacrifice its damaged proteins and old or sick cells (such as cancer cells) first. Immune cells will tag damaged proteins and old, sick and cancerous cells, and those cells will be digested and recycled back into new cells and tissues. As a result, you're fighting the main cause of aging, which is the failure of your body to repair or replace damaged cells. This doesn't mean the aging process stops; but this process does slow down the proliferation of damaged or aged cells in your body.

During the same above-referenced study in 2011, researchers at the Intermountain Medical Center Heart Institute found the following:

> This recent study also confirmed earlier findings about the effects of fasting on human growth hormone (HGH), a metabolic protein. HGH works to protect lean muscle and metabolic balance, a response triggered and accelerated by fasting. During the 24-hour fasting periods, HGH increased an average of 1,300 percent in women and nearly 2,000 percent in men.

We now know that healthy levels of HGH are important to the anti-aging process. You may have seen commercials peddling HGH level-optimizing supplements recently, because some companies know the importance of HGH as well. Now, that's not to say certain natural-based supplements can't be used to assist with HGH levels; however, most of the ones you see advertised, making outrageous health claims, are pure junk. I can guarantee you won't lose drastic weight and gain hard, lean muscle by taking their magical health supplement.

MY INTERMITTENT FASTING TIPS FOR SUCCESS

1. Work your way up to the 16-hour fast. First try going four or five hours between meals, and then increase that amount gradually.

2. Remember, you naturally go into fat-burning mode while you sleep; this is the reason you fast from your last meal in the evening until the 14 to 16-hour mark is reached the next day. The main concept of intermittent fasting is to prolong the natural fat-burning mode that occurs during your sleep cycle.

3. Coconut oil is your friend during fasting. It's comprised of medium-chain triglycerides, which are easily converted into ketone bodies and have a glycemic index of 0 (all healthy fats have a 0 glycemic index). Thus, there's no insulin response but plenty of quick energy.

4. If you feel lightheaded during your fast, eat something. This could mean your blood glucose is extremely low (hypoglycemic).

5. If you're pregnant, or trying to conceive, you shouldn't use fasting techniques.

6. Yes, it's safe for athletes to use intermittent fasting; you won't bonk if fully fat-adapted. I often road or mountain bike for several hours without carb-loading or sucking down packs of sugar filled goo—just water is sufficient. But being a competitive athlete has far different macro-nutrient requirements than the everyday Joe and Jane, so you'll have to experiment and adapt to your own level of training.

17

The Simple Life Healthy Lifestyle
Starter Grocery Shopping List

Here's *The Simple Life Healthy Lifestyle* starter grocery shopping list to help you get started on your path to optimal health (sign up for my updates and get this as a free download).

Note that all of the oils, herbs and spices should be organic, and the oils should be cold-pressed and virgin. It's not essential for your fruits, vegetables, dairy and meats to be all organic or free-range right away, though, because I want you to get comfortable making better choices and figuring out where to purchase these items.

In the beginning, changing your shopping habits can be difficult, but I'd like you to start incorporating organic and free-range products into your lifestyle as soon as possible. The end goal is for you to not only be eating, but also living, a Primal lifestyle. That comes with purchasing the healthiest organic foods possible (or even better, growing and raising your own).

Note: I've put (organic) next to the items that I feel are the most important to purchase this way in the beginning.

Fats and Oils (*organic*)

Coconut oil (*for high-heat cooking*)
Palm oil (*for high-heat cooking/frying*)
Olive oil (*for drizzling*)
Butter (*for medium-heat cooking*)

Herbs and Spices (*organic*)

Basil
Cilantro
Cinnamon
Cumin
Turmeric
Celtic sea salt
Himalayan salt
Nutmeg
Garlic
Ginger
Black Pepper

Nuts

Macadamia nuts
Brazil nuts
Almonds
Pecans

Grain Flour Replacements

Coconut flour
Almond flour

Meat and Poultry

Beef

Bison (buffalo)

Lamb

Chicken (also eggs)

Pork

Turkey

Duck (also eggs)

Remember to include organ meats

Seafood (*wild-caught*)

Salmon

Trout

Cod

Mahi mahi

Tuna

Anchovies

Sardines

Scallops

Shrimp

Clams

Dairy (*organic*)

Kefir

Cheese

Whole milk

Cottage cheese

Vegetables

Avocados

Broccoli

Tomatoes

Spinach

Kale

Mushrooms

Onions

Romaine lettuce

Squash

Olives

Cucumbers

Cauliflower

Carrots

Garlic

Cabbage

Fruits

Best for Weight Loss

Blackberries

Blueberries

Raspberries

Cranberries

Other Acceptable Fruits

Bananas

Apples

Cherries

Coconut

Lemons
Limes
Oranges
Peaches
Pears
Pineapple
Plums
Strawberries
Pomegranate
Watermelon

Beverages
Water (*filtered*)
Tea (*organic*)
Coffee (*organic*)
Coconut milk
Almond milk

Sweeteners
Stevia
Xylitol (*Note: Be careful with sugar alcohols—they can cause bloating and digestive issues for some, especially when too much is consumed*)
Local raw honey (*in moderation*)
Maple syrup (*in moderation*)
Coconut sugar (*in moderation*)

Sauces and Condiments

Coconut aminos (*as a substitute for soy sauce*)

Mustard (*all types*)

Hot sauce (*gluten-free*)

Ketchup (*organic, in moderation*)

Salsa

Green chiles

Guacamole

Supplements

The Simple Life Organic Greens Powder

The Simple Life Turmeric

The Simple Life Vitamin D3

The Simple Life Fish Oil (Omega 3)

The Simple Life Probiotics

The Simple Life Men's/Women's Daily Multi-Vitamin

The above supplements are available at **www.thesimplelifenow. com**. You can also get all of them in a convenient discounted package on *The Simple Life* website.

18

The Simple Life Healthy Lifestyle Starter Recipes

SOME COOKING BASICS

I'll now discuss some basic ingredients that you'll need in order to get started, and some basic guidelines to make your healthy cooking transition easier.

Herbs and Spices

Here are some basic herbs and spices for you to purchase and use. Feel free to experiment, as we all have our different tastes and preferences. As you become more comfortable, add more and more herbs and spices to your menu options, or simply keep it basic. I personally only use a couple of herbs and spices regularly. They can be fresh (preferably) or dried.

- Celtic sea salt (*remember, you can safely use two to two-and-a-half teaspoons of natural salt a day in your foods*)

- Himalayan salt

- Basil

- Cayenne

- Black Pepper

- Garlic

- Cilantro

- Cinnamon

- Nutmeg

- Stevia

- Turmeric

Core Oils

When it come to oils, in the beginning it's best to keep it simple. Make sure they're virgin, cold-pressed and organic. Remember that when vegetable oils are highly processed—as are most commercially available vegetable oils today—they have likely become rancid. Rancid oils will have the opposite effect of healthy oils, which means they'll cause inflammation and free radicals in the body instead of providing the life-giving properties of healthy oils.

- Coconut oil (*use for cooking at higher heats*)

- Palm oil (*use for frying, as it's a very stable oil at high heat*)

- Butter (*use only organic butter; best for cooking at low to medium temps*)

- Olive oil (*can be used for medium-heat cooking, but I recommend using it for drizzling on salads and vegetables instead. It's easy to overheat olive oil to the point of turning it rancid.*)

I call these the core oils because I consider them to be the healthiest and the most easy-to-find oils in stores. When it comes to cooking with virgin coconut oil, it will take a little time to get used to, as it has a slight coconut and vanilla flavor. It's the oil that is most stable, though. And it contains lauric acid, which is an incredibly strong antimicrobial component, thus helping to boost your immune system.

Organic is Always Best

Remember to always use organic ingredients when possible, as they are, by far, the better choice. If you have the time and space, I highly recommend that you grow your own organic garden and use your own fruits and vegetables. I don't go into organics too much in this book, as they're a whole topic on their own. With that being said, try to use as many organic products as you can. It may take a while to find them, but add them in as you can and get yourself more comfortable with organic foods.

Throw Away the Plastic

If there's one last piece of important health advice I can give you, it's to get rid of all your plastic storage containers. Plastic is a curse from the "poison-you-slowly" gods! Most, if not all, plastics leach chemicals into the food they're storing, including BPA (Bisphenol A), a known endocrine (hormone) mimicker and disrupter. Throw in the fact that most plastic food containers are made in China, which is notorious for flouting manufacturing regulations, and you have a noxious chemical storing device best kept out of your home. The fix is simple: Just replace the plastic with glass storage containers, and try to find ones made in the USA. *Pyrex* is the most common brand and can be found at almost any retail store. They're very inexpensive and will last a lifetime if taken care of properly.

Homemade = Savings!

Home-cooked meals are far cheaper than their chemical- and preservative-stuffed relatives at most fast-food or chain restaurants. On average, the meals in this guide will cost you less than $2 to prepare yourself. Even when choosing the dollar (that is, no-nutrition) menu, it's a struggle to eat out for less than $5 to $10. But preparing your food at home can save you 80 percent or more; I have clients regularly save thousands of dollars a year by cooking their own healthy organic meals.

If you eat lunch out on a daily basis, that equals about 130 days a year. That means you're spending somewhere in the neighborhood of $1,300 a year on just one meal a day! Cooking your own meals and bringing them with you for lunch will cost you under $300 a year. I eat pretty much a 100 percent organic diet and the cost is nowhere near what I'd spend if I ate my meals out like most Americans do today. The best part is I save a ton of money, not only on food but on doctor's visits as well!

One thing some of you will notice in the recipes that follow is the absence of precise measurements. There's a good reason for this: Even though most meals in this guide yield one serving, I like to go by taste when measuring. I've created some phenomenal new recipes by doing this. Plus, I believe in freedom of food choice and not eating the exact same thing every time. You'll also notice, as you revert back to a more natural eating approach, that organic and real food varies in taste from batch to batch, crop to crop. That being said, you'll need to test out your measurements and see what works best for you. For that matter, you may not want to use some of the ingredients outlined in my recipes. Wow! Food freedom, here we come!

Breakfast

I love breakfast! As a matter of fact, I eat breakfast for lunch and dinner some days, as it's what I consider the simplest and quickest meal to prepare. There's nothing wrong with eating a meal that most would consider breakfast a couple of times a day. Remember, those ingrained standard American meals are the old way we look at food. Now we look at food with a new pair of traditional diet lenses. Do you think our distant ancestors would have always had meals specifically categorized every day? No, they would have eaten what they had at hand, or what was abundant to hunt or gather at the time. Don't be afraid to be different and break the mold. If you feel like eating a certain type of food for a day, such as if you find yourself craving eggs, go for it. More than likely that craving is your body telling you it's deficient in one of the micro or macronutrients contained in that food.

You'll also notice these recipes are gluten-free for the most part, depending on which of the ingredients you use. For those who have a gluten intolerance or allergy, or who have celiac disease, these are great alternatives. For those who have no problems with gluten or grains, feel free to substitute the grain products of your choice. Remember, we don't prescribe one food type for all but encourage a more well-rounded approach, as everyone has different ancestry, dietary needs and tolerances.

Make It Simple Breakfast

- 2 whole eggs, prepared the way you want (*over-easy, scrambled, etc.*)

- Chopped onion, as much as you want

- Spinach, as much as you want

- A small serving of diced sweet potato

- (*Optional*) A couple of links of sausage or slices of bacon (*organic, if possible*)

1. *Put one to two teaspoons of coconut oil in a cast iron or stainless steel frying pan (no non-stick pans, as they leach chemicals into your food) and let it melt before putting any food in the pan.*

2. *Cook your sweet potato first, as it takes the longest to cook.*

3. *If you're scrambling your eggs, cook your onions and spinach first before mixing them in with the eggs.*

4. *Cook your eggs (mix in your pre-cooked onions and spinach if you're scrambling)*

5. *If your optional meat choice is pre-cooked, which most sausage is today, you'll have to determine the best time to prepare it so it's done at the same time as the other parts of your meal.*

For those of you who haven't cooked very much, or who've only cooked infrequently, this may seem like a daunting meal to prepare. The first couple of times you'll have to experiment, but trust me, once you get it down you can knock this meal out in about five to ten minutes. Quick and healthy, that's what we're going for!

Gary's Go-Gurt

- 4 to 6 ounces of Greek-style plain yogurt or kefir (*if you have problems with dairy, use a dairy alternative such as an almond- or coconut-based yogurt*)

- Cinnamon, to taste

- Stevia or a small amount of natural sugar, to taste

- A small handful of berries, such as blueberries, raspberries or blackberries

Put everything in a bowl, mix together and, boom, *breakfast is served.*

This is also a great on-the-go meal you can take with you. I love this breakfast, which can also be used as a snack, because you can find these food items anywhere and they don't require any cooking.

Gary's Get Up and Get Going Protein Shake

- 1 to 2 scoops of *The Simple Life* brand or other high-quality protein powder of your choice

- ½ a frozen banana

- A couple of dashes of cinnamon

- A dash of nutmeg

- 1 to 2 teaspoons of almond butter

- 8 to 10 ounces of coconut or almond milk

- Water, if needed, to get the consistency you desire

Mix all ingredients in a blender until they're amalgamated with no clumps.

Note: I prefer to mix my protein shakes in a stainless steel old-style milkshake mixer container when using a hand blender. That way I don't have to worry about plastic leaching or fragments from the blending process getting into my protein shake. You can find these shake blender containers at restaurant specialty stores on the Internet. They're a little pricey, but I've had mine for several years and it will more than likely outlast me. I'm a big fan of buying products that are not only healthy, but can be used for a lifetime.

This is one of the quickest meals to prepare and take with you, and it can be consumed any time of the day. Often while on the road or traveling to appointments, I'll pack a protein shake with me so I have a healthy meal and won't be tempted to buy something from the gas station or grab-and-dash mini-market.

Gary's Primal Breakfast

- 2 teaspoons of coconut oil or butter

- Pre-cooked steak, diced (*a great way to use leftover steak*)

- 2 whole eggs, prepared the way you like them

- 1 tomato, diced

- ½ an avocado, diced

- (*Optional*) Cheese of your choice, to be mixed in with the eggs if scrambling

1. *Pre-heat your frying pan with the oil or butter.*

2. *Warm up the pre-cooked steak first, separately from the eggs.*

3. *Cook your eggs (you can mix in the tomatoes and avocado if scrambling, or put those on top if frying).*

When I cook a steak, I usually can't eat the entire piece as most cuts are too big for my preference. So I'll use whatever's left over for breakfast the next morning. When reheated in coconut oil or butter, it tastes fantastic!

Coconut Flour Pancakes

When it comes to pancakes and other breakfast flour-based products, use caution. First, a large number of people have difficulties digesting grains, and second, grain-based products are loaded with empty carbohydrates. I'm a big fan of using grain-free alternative flours to avoid the above issues. You must remember, though, that these grain replacements still contain carbs, so make sure not to overdo it.

I don't give precise measurements here, since I like to mix the batter to the best consistency and taste. You'll have to experiment to find what works best for you. Note that the pancake mixture should be fairly thick in order to produce nice, fluffy cakes.

- Oil or butter of your choice

- 2 whole eggs

- ½ a cup of coconut flour (*start here and and add more, if needed, to get the proper consistency*)

- ½ teaspoon of cinnamon (*add more to taste, if needed*)

- A couple of dashes of nutmeg, to taste

- 2 pinches of sea salt

- 1 to 2 tablespoons of almond butter (*this will make the 'cakes nutty and moist*)

- Stevia, if needed to get the desired sweetness

- Coconut milk (*add until the desired consistency is reached*)

- (*Optional*) Vanilla extract, to taste

- (*Optional*) Strawberries, blueberries or raspberries, diced

1. *Mix all of your ingredients together in a large mixing bowl until all lumps are gone and you have a smooth consistency.*

2. *Pour your pancake batter, to the size you desire, into a medium heated, oiled stainless steel or cast iron pan, and cook until lightly browned on both sides.*

Here's a great way to add flavor to your pancakes: Use the grease from any sausage or bacon that will accompany your meal to cook your pancakes in. If you don't want to use bacon or sausage grease, use coconut oil, butter or palm oil to cook them in.

For your toppings, use fruit, real maple syrup, yogurt or, one of my favorites, melted honey and butter.

These pancakes are not low-carb, but they're far healthier than the garbage mixes they sell in the grocery store, and better yet, they're gluten-free!

Lunch

For most people, lunch is the toughest meal of the day, as most Americans are at work or on the go during this time. I have found when working with clients that, by just changing their lunch eating habits, we can make huge strides to getting them on track. The easiest way to deal with poor lunch choices while at work or on the road is to pack a protein shake. Not only is it a far healthier choice, but depending on where you usually purchase that health-killing meal, it can cost between 80 to 90 percent less than the average American lunch out. Wow, talk about a win-win situation: better health and saving loads of money!

The Healthy Hunter's Protein Shake

- 1 to 2 scoops of *The Simple Life* brand or other high-quality protein powder of your choice

- ½ a cup of frozen raspberries or strawberries

- 1 to 2 teaspoons of almond butter

- 8 to 10 ounces of coconut or almond milk

- Add water, if needed, to get the consistency you desire

Mix with a blender or hand blender until all the ingredients are fully combined and there are no clumps.

I kid you not, it's that simple! People are amazed at how quick and easy this lunch or meal-on-the-go solution is.

Bonus hint: After blending your protein shake, put it in the freezer for 15 minutes prior to leaving your house and it will stay cold until lunchtime.

The Omnivore's (No) Dilemma Salad

Salads are some of the easiest, quickest and healthiest meal choices. Here's one of my favorite recipes that you can take with you in a sealed container to work.

- 1 cup of your favorite leafy vegetable or greens mix, such as kale, spinach, romaine or a combination of all three

- A handful of almonds

- 1 to 2 tablespoons of goat cheese

- ¼ cup of carrots, shredded

- ½ a medium size tomato, diced

- 4 to 6 ounces of shredded or diced cooked chicken

- A drizzle of olive oil or red wine vinaigrette, to taste

- A pinch of sea salt, if so desired

Mix the first six ingredients together in a bowl, then add the vinaigrette and salt to taste.

I consider this my quick-and-dirty lunch meal choice as I can make it in mere minutes. I've taken this lunch staple with me to the office for decades and, just like the shake, it's quick and doesn't kill the pocketbook. This same salad in a restaurant can cost $10 to $12. Your cost, by making it yourself, is under $2.

Gary's Triple-P (Power, Protein and Pasta)

- ½ a cup of cooked full-fat ground turkey or beef (*free-range or grass-fed, if you can find it*)

- ½ a cup of grain-free or gluten-free pasta

- Marinara sauce

- 2 tablespoons of shredded cheese of your choice

1. *Brown the ground turkey or beef in a frying pan and season to your preference.*

2. *Cook the pasta to your preference in a pot of boiling water. (Note: If you're going to take this to lunch with you, it's better to cook the pasta to an al dente texture, which means still firm but not hard. If you cook it more than this, you risk it being mushy if eaten as a leftover.)*

3. *Combine the pasta and ground meat, then mix in some warmed marinara sauce, but don't drown it. (Note: Almost all tomato-based sauces contain added sugar unless you make them yourself, so be sure to check the label on your sauce.)*

4. *Top with the shredded cheese.*

Low-carb doesn't mean you can't ever eat pasta again! The great thing about a meal like this, and others like it, is that you don't have to reheat it if you're in a pinch. You will notice my lunch choices are very portable and most can be eaten cold.

I'm Hungry Now Shrimp Dish

- ½ a cup of peeled zucchini or other squash (*use a potato peeler or spiralizer to get pasta-like strips*)

- Butter, to cook the squash in

- ½ a cup of cooked shrimp

- ¼ cup of fresh cilantro, chopped

- Basil-based salad dressing

- Sea salt, to taste

1. *Cook your squash in a frying pan with butter.*

2. *Add the shrimp and cilantro to your cooked squash and mix together.*

3. *Drizzle on some basil-based dressing or just olive oil.*

4. *Top with a pinch or two of sea salt.*

This is about as simple as it gets and, trust me, this meal is absolutely yummy! It's just as good hot as cold, and is a great dinner idea as well.

The Guiltless Wrap

I prefer to use a coconut flour-based wrap to stay gluten-free. But you can use lettuce as your wrap, or something else low-carb.

- 1 wrap of your choice

- Lunch meat of your choice

- ½ a medium avocado, diced

- 2 tablespoons of shredded cheddar cheese

- ½ a medium size tomato, diced

1. *Using a wrap of your choice, add a few slices of good quality, non-nitrate/nitrite lunch meat or, better yet, use leftover meat that you've prepared earlier.*

2. *Add the avocado, cheese (remember, raw milk and organic is best), and tomato.*

3. *Wrap that bad boy up and you're ready to go!*

Dinner

Gary's Simple Stir Fry

People are constantly amazed at how easy this meal is to prepare. As a matter of fact, once I show people this little gem, it's often all they'll eat for several days in a row because it's so easy to prepare yet tastes great. The different variants of this dish are limitless—use your imagination, as you can substitute a multitude of other ingredients.

- 2 to 3 tablespoons of coconut oil

- ½ to 1 pound of your favorite raw meat, cut into cubes

- 1 medium size green or yellow squash, sliced thinly or diced (*whichever you prefer*)

- ¼ of a medium size yellow onion, diced

- 1 whole tomato, diced

- 1 to 2 tablespoons of coconut aminos or gluten-free soy sauce

- (*Optional*) Fresh basil and/or cilantro, to taste

- (*Optional*) Sea salt

1. *On medium to high heat, melt the coconut oil in a large frying pan.*

2. *Brown your cubed meat, then add all of the vegetables except the tomatoes.*

3. *Stir for 2 to 3 minutes, then add the tomatoes.*

4. *Add the coconut aminos or soy sauce.*

5, *If you'd like, add some fresh basil, cilantro or both.*

6. *If needed, add sea salt to your taste preference.*

You'll have to test and experiment with how you like your vegetables cooked. I like mine to be slightly cooked and still a little raw, but that's my preference. Also, if you add the tomatoes earlier they'll come out almost stewed, which will change the texture and flavor.

Gary's Crazy (as in Darn Good!) Sausage Goulash

This is one of my all-time favorites as it's incredibly simple, quick and great tasting.

- 2 tablespoons of coconut oil

- 1 cup of frozen or fresh carrots, broccoli and cauliflower

- 8-to-10-inch link of organic or high-quality sausage

- Coconut aminos or gluten-free soy sauce, to taste

- Sea salt, to taste

1. *Melt the coconut oil in a large frying pan.*

2. *Once the oil is melted, add the vegetables and cook at medium heat until they start to soften.*

3. *Cut the sausage into round slices, to the thickness of your choice, and add them to the pan.*

4. *Stir until cooked to your preference, then drizzle in a little coconut aminos or gluten-free soy sauce.*

5. *Add sea salt if needed.*

Just like that, dinner is served! This is a wonderful dish for when you're in a hurry but still want to eat a tremendously healthy meal. Feel free to mix it up—I'll sometimes add turmeric, cilantro or basil, depending on what I have on hand and how much time I have.

Gary's Ground Meat Spectacular

This is another one of my favorites, as it's super quick and makes for some really good leftovers.

- 1 pound of full-fat ground turkey or ground beef (*free-range or grass-fed, if you can find it*)

- Spices of your preference

- ½ a cup of carrots, diced

- ½ a cup of squash, diced

- ¼ to ½ of a medium size onion, diced

- Tomato sauce, such as marinara sauce

1. *Defrost the ground meat if it's frozen.*

2. *Begin to brown the meat in a large frying pan, adding spices of your choice. I prefer to use turmeric and sea salt, but good alternatives are garlic powder, basil, chili powder, etc.*

3. *Once the meat is about halfway cooked, add the diced vegetables and stir from time to time to cook food consistently.*

4. *Add some type of tomato sauce, such as marinara sauce, but only a little. Mix in until the meat and vegetables are lightly coated.*

That's all there is to it! You now have your main course—or sometimes I'll eat it as my only course for the day. It has everything you need: protein, vegetables and fat, and is a quick power meal in just minutes!

Stick It With a Stick Skewers

For anyone who loves to barbeque, this is another simple and great dinner idea. You'll need some steel skewers or the disposable wood version.

- 1 pound of raw meat of your choice

- Coconut aminos or gluten-free soy sauce

- Red and green bell peppers, cut into chunks

- Onions, cut into chunks

- (*Optional*) White rice

1. *Cube up roughly a pound of meat of your choice, such as chicken, fish, lamb or beef.*

2. *I like to marinate my meat for about an hour before I cook it. The easiest way to do that is to simply pour about ¼-inch of coconut aminos into one of your new glass food storage containers, put your meat in, put the lid on (tight and sealed, otherwise you'll be cursing) and shake it every fifteen minutes. After about an hour, it's nice and tender and ready to go.*

3. *Cut up some bell peppers and onions to a good size so they won't fall off the skewers.*

4. *Place your meat and vegetable chunks onto the steel or wood skewers, alternating them until the skewers are filled up.*

5. *Pre-heat your barbecue and cook until done.*

6. *Pull the meat and vegetables off the skewers and onto a plate and dig in.*

You can eat these alone as a meal, but I like to have them on a small bed of white rice.

Chicken Fingers Lickin' Good

This is another super easy meal that's a family favorite and also one of mine.

- Coconut or palm oil (*enough to submerge at least half of the meat you'll be deep-frying*)

- Raw, boneless chicken or turkey (*free-range is best*)

- 2 to 4 whole eggs

- Coconut flour

- Sea salt

- Spices of your choice

1. *Portion up some chicken or turkey into nuggets.*

2. *Put the eggs in a mixing bowl and whisk until the yolks and whites are fully blended together.*

3. *Prepare a bowl of coconut flour, as you'll be breading the nuggets with this. I like to add sea salt, but you can add pepper and other spices of your choice to the breading flour. (Note: You can also use or add a whole grain of your choice, but I like to make these grain-free by using only coconut flour.)*

4. *Preheat (medium to high heat) a large frying pan and melt the coconut or palm oil.*

5. *Dunk each nugget into the mixed eggs until the entire nugget is coated.*

6. *Roll the egg-covered nugget in the bowl of flour until it's fully covered.*

7. *Now you're ready to do some frying. Carefully place the breaded nuggets into the hot oil. (**Warning: Do not use a bare, uncovered hand to do this. Instead, use a utensil long enough to keep your hand and body away from the heated oil. You can get severely burned by splattering oil when placing meat in a hot pan.**)*

8. *Fry the nuggets until golden brown on both sides, then remove from the pan, once again using caution.*

Get out of here, McDonald's! We have chicken nuggets that actually contain chicken!

I like to prepare a simple salad as my side dish, but any vegetables of your choice make a good complementary food for these healthy nuggets.

Filling in the Gaps

Now that we have the major meals covered, it's time to fill in the gaps with some healthy go-anywhere snacks. Many people struggle when that 2 to 3 p.m. window hits at work, and they're tempted to go the vending machine and purchase some insidious packaged snack. Since I've spent a large part of my life traveling for work, or on-the-go, I've developed some really easy, healthy snack choices to have instead.

Nuts, Nuts, Where are my Nuts?!

Nuts are such an incredibly easy snack. I always have some in a bag at home, or in a sealed container in my computer bag. They can take heat, cold and a lot of abuse, making them the ultimate snack for on-the-go. Not just any type of nut will do, though.

I have two choices that I consider to be the healthiest and most appealing to palates: almonds and macadamia nuts. I prefer them in the organic raw version, but some people like them better roasted. Either option is a good choice, but almonds are usually about half the price of macadamia nuts, so your pocketbook could be the final determinant. And don't feel that you can only eat these two choices—feel free to mix it up from time to time.

Note that peanuts are not nuts, they are actually beans (legumes). For numerous reasons, I recommend using alternatives other than peanuts, but if you like them I don't completely discourage people from consuming them.

You can also get creative and make your own trail mix. Most trail mixes in the store are loaded with sugar, so I would recommend you stay away from these sugar bombs disguised as a healthy choice.

Remember, though, don't go nuts for nuts. They're meant to be used as a snack, not a meal substitute.

Apples

I like apples as a good snack because of their durability and shelf life. The hardcore diet gurus might say that they're too high on the glycemic index, and they're not entirely wrong. If you're trying to lose weight, other fruit choices (like berries) are better. But when you're on the go, an apple is not going to hurt you or make you gain five pounds on the spot.

With all fruits, especially the higher sugar-content variety, I recommend you never eat them by themselves. I suggest you combine fruit with a food high in a good healthy fat, such as nuts or cheese. This will slow down the sugar absorbed into your bloodstream, thus avoiding those dreaded insulin spikes. The good news is that fruits naturally have a good amount of fiber so they automatically slow the absorption of glucose into your bloodstream, as compared to unnatural sugary snacks.

I recommend apples because of their durability factor, but a small amount of fruit is always a great snack choice. Berries are especially good because they contain high amounts of antioxidants and are lower in sugar than other fruits.

Protein Shakes

These are an incredibly efficient way to consume something healthier than the usual fast food while on the go.

Hardboiled Eggs

I picked these little gems because they're easy to make and pretty durable. I also consider eggs to be one of the best foods you can eat in order to be healthy—they pack a big nutrient punch in a small package. When I need a quick snack, I chomp down two hardboiled eggs and I'm good to go!

Desserts

Now let's move on to everyone's favorite: desserts! As I discuss in my numerous articles, being healthy doesn't mean you can never eat anything sweet again. What it does mean is you need to make smart choices when it comes to sweets, and you must make them yourself. There are very few, if any, pre-packaged desserts that aren't loaded with sugar. Worse yet, they're also usually loaded with highly processed ingredients.

Some make the mistake of just trading in their processed sugar treats for more natural sugar treats, expecting better health results. They're always greatly disappointed when pretty much nothing changes, though. Remember, an organically made cookie is still a cookie!

Now let's look at some healthier sweet alternatives I've come up with over the years that allow us to follow *The Simple Life Healthy Lifestyle Plan*.

Gary's White Clouds of Heaven

- The whites of 2 eggs (*separated from the yolks*)

- Stevia (*and cinnamon, if you want*), to taste

- Fresh fruit (*I've noticed that blueberries are an excellent choice with this dessert*)

1. *Put the egg whites in a small to medium mixing bowl and, using an electric mixer or whisk, mix until fluffy.*

2. *Add stevia (and cinnamon, if you want), to taste.*

3. *Continue to mix until the egg whites hold a stiff shape when you take the mixing utensil out of the bowl. The egg white mixture should look like a mountain peak, but of sweet joy!*

4. *Transfer the mixture to a normal eating bowl and add fresh fruit of your choice.*

Pretty simple and incredibly healthy!

Guiltless Homemade Chocolate

- Equal amounts of coconut oil and cocoa butter (*Note: the cocoa butter you're looking for is not suntan lotion—it can be found in many health food stores and is a yellowish, solid-looking fat*)

- Real cocoa or cacao powder

- 1 teaspoon of vanilla extract

- Stevia, to taste (*if you prefer a low-sugar version*)

- (*Optional*) 1 to 2 tablespoons of unsalted butter

- (*Optional*) Real maple syrup instead of stevia

- (*Optional*) Carob powder, to taste

- (*Optional*) A pinch or two of sea salt

1. *Into a saucepan (the size should be determined by the amount of chocolate you're making), place equal amounts of coconut oil and cocoa butter.*

2. *On low heat, melt the coconut oil and cocoa butter together (the slower the better—don't let it get to a boil).*

3. *Once the ingredients are completely melted, take the pot off the heat and mix in the cocoa or cacao powder. (Note: It may take a couple of batches for you to get the flavor just how you like it—there's no magic formula—but it should look dark and somewhat creamy. Also, melted homemade real chocolate is runnier than store-bought chocolate.)*

4. *Mix in the vanilla extract.*

5. *Add stevia, to taste, if you prefer a low-sugar version. Or use real maple syrup, to your preferred taste.*

6. *(Optional) Melt in 1 to 2 tablespoons of real unsalted butter.*

7. *(Optional) Mix in some carob powder; I often do this.*

8. *(Optional) Mix in a pinch or two of sea salt.*

9. *Make sure all of the ingredients are well mixed. Use only a spoon to combine (no power mixers are needed) and keep the chocolate in the saucepan until the end.*

10. *Now let the mixture cool to room temperature. Once at room temperature, make any last-minute adjustments to adjust the the taste to your preference.*

11. *Place the saucepan in your refrigerator and cover it with a lid, or pour it into a glass baking dish and cover it with some type of wrap. Then check on it every 5 to 10 minutes until the chocolate mixture solidifies. I like to mix it with a spoon two to three times until it starts to thicken, as the oils tend to separate.*

12. *Once the mixture is solid—usually in about 20 to 30 minutes—break it up and put the pieces in a glass container. Real chocolate has a lower melting temperature than processed store-bought chocolate, so you'll have to store it in the refrigerator at all times.*

Gary's Gluten-Free Gooey Cookies

- 2 cups of almond flour or coconut flour

- ¼ teaspoon baking soda

- ¼ teaspoon sea salt

- ½ a cup of honey

- ⅓ cup of coconut

- (Optional) Stevia

- 1 teaspoon vanilla extract

- Guiltless Homemade Chocolate or store-bought chocolate chips

1. *Preheat oven to 350° F (160° C).*

2. *Combine the almond or coconut flour with the baking soda and sea salt in a large bowl and mix together until fully combined.*

3. *Melt the honey and coconut oil together in a small saucepan. (Optional: Use stevia in place of honey to reduce the sugar content. If you do this, though, you'll need to add more coconut oil to keep it moist.)*

4. *Once the honey (or stevia) and oil are melted, add the vanilla extract.*

5. *Combine the melted ingredients with the dry ingredients and mix until no clumps are present.*

6. Using the homemade chocolate recipe above, add in small bits of chocolate and mix again. (Optional: Use store-bought, pre-made chocolate chips instead.)

7. Using a tablespoon or cookie dough scoop, scoop out even amounts of dough and roll into balls.

8. Place the dough balls, evenly spaced, on a lined baking tray (parchment paper or Silpat sheets work well), then bake them for 10 to 12 minutes. (Note: If you like them gooier, cook them for less time.)

Gary's Greatest Almond Butter

(*In order to make this, you'll need a Vitamix or similar heavy-duty blender.*)

- 1 pound of raw almonds

- 2 tablespoons of coconut oil

- 4 to 5 pinches of sea salt

- (*Optional*) 1 teaspoon of ground cinnamon

1. *Preheat oven to 350° F (160° C).*

2. *Place the raw almonds on a cookie sheet and bake for 5 to 10 minutes. (Note: Every batch of raw almonds is different, as the size and water content will vary. It will take anywhere from 5 to 10 minutes to bake your almonds, and the length of time you bake them will change the flavor of your almond butter. For a darker, richer flavor, bake them a little longer, being careful not to burn them.)*

3. *Take the almonds out of the oven and let them cool to room temperature on the cookie sheet.*

4. *Once cooled, put all of the almonds into your Vitamix (or similar) blender.*

5. *Add the coconut oil (I like to pour it into the middle of the almonds as I add them to the blender).*

6. *Add 4 to 5 pinches of sea salt.*

7. *(Optional) Add 1 teaspoon of ground cinnamon.*

8. *Now you're ready to start mixing. This is where it becomes an art form: The faster you grind the almonds, the more liquid your almond butter will be. I like to mix mine using the lower power setting with the dial set at 7 (if using a Vitamix). You'll have to experiment to get it to the texture you prefer, though.*

9. *Once you get the consistency you like, simply scoop your nut butter out of the blender with a small batter spatula.*

10. *Store your almond butter in a glass container in the refrigerator, as this is a natural product with no preservatives. It will usually stay good for a couple of weeks, although mine never lasts that long because I eat it all!*

Note: The reason you bake the almonds is that you need to weaken the cell walls in order to get the oil out. If you don't do this, you'll just make almond flour when you blend them together. *Bonus:* Now you know how to make your own almond flour as well!

Here's the best part: You can change the flavor of your almond butter by simply changing the length of the almond baking time, and change the consistency by varying the speed at which you grind the nuts.

You may be asking, how is almond butter a dessert? It may not be one technically, but I'll tell you, after a couple of spoons of almond butter, my sweet tooth is usually taken care of.

Also, if you put it on some banana or apple slices, it's pure heaven!

Low-Sugar/Dairy-Free Ice Cream

(*In order to make this, you'll need a Vitamix or similar heavy-duty blender. The blending instructions below are specifically for a Vitamix, but you can modify them to fit your blender if using another brand.*)

- 1 cup of coconut milk

- 1 cup of ice

- 1 pound of strawberries or other fruit of your choice (*to keep the glycemic level lowest, use berries of any type*)

- 1 teaspoon vanilla extract

- 1 teaspoon cinnamon

- (*Optional*) Stevia, to desired sweetness

1. *Put all of the ingredients into a Vitamix (or similar) blender.*

1. *Select variable 1.*

2. *Turn the machine on and quickly increase the speed to variable 10, then to high.*

3. *Use the tamper to press the ingredients into the blades.*

4. *In about 30 to 60 seconds, the sound of the motor will change and four mounds should form.*

5. *Stop the machine. Do not overmix or melting will occur.*

6. *Scoop the mixture into a bowl and serve immediately.*

Did You Enjoy This Book? You Can Make a Big Difference and Spread the Word!

Reviews are the most powerful tool I have to bring attention to *The Simple Life*. I'm an independently published author and yes, I do a lot of this work myself. This helps me make sure the information I provide is straight from the heart and comes from my experiences without some publishing company dictating what sells. You, the readers, are my muscle and marketing machine.

You are a committed group and a loyal bunch of fans!

I truly love my fans and the passion they have for my writing and products. Simply put, your reviews help bring more fans to my books and attention to what I'm trying to teach.

If you liked this book, or any of my others for that matter, I would be very grateful if you would spend a couple of minutes and leave a review. Doesn't have to be long, just something conveying your thoughts.

Please visit Amazon.com to leave a review for my book(s).

Thank you!

Get Your Free Goodies and Stuff!

Building a solid relationship with my readers is very important to me. It is one of the rewards of being a writer. From time to time, I send out my newsletter (never spammy, I promise) to keep you up to date with special offers and information about anything new I may be doing.

If that's not enough enticement, when you sign up for my newsletter I'll send you some spectacular free stuff!

1. Gary's three-day fat blast

2. Gary's current workout routine

3. Beginner grocery shopping list

You can get all the goodies above by signing up for my mailing list at: **www.thesimplelifenow.com/healthyresources**.

ABOUT GARY

Gary Collins, MS, was raised in the High Desert at the basin of the Sierra Nevada mountain range in a rural part of California. He now lives part of the year in a remote area of northeast Washington State, and the other part of the year is dedicated to exploring in his travel trailer with his trusty black lab Barney.

Gary considers himself lucky to have grown up in a very small town experiencing fishing, hunting, and anything outdoors from a very young age. He has been involved in organized sports, nutrition, and fitness for almost four decades. He is also an active follower and teacher of what he calls "life simplification." He believes that *"Today we're bombarded by too much stress, and not enough time for personal fulfillment. We're failing to take care of our health and be truly happy...there has to be a better way!"*

Collins' background is very unique and brings a much-needed perspective to today's conversations about health, nutrition, entrepreneurship, self-help and self-reliance. He holds an AS degree in Exercise Science, a BS in Criminal Justice, and an MS in Forensic Science.

He has a unique and interesting background that includes military intelligence, and roles as a special agent for the U.S. State Department Diplomatic Security Service, the U.S. Department of Health and Human Services, and the U.S. Food and Drug Administration.

In addition to being a best-selling author, Gary has taught at the university level, consulted and trained college-level athletes, and been interviewed for his expertise on various subjects by *CBS Sports, Coast to Coast AM, The RT Network*, and *FOX News* to name a few.

The Simple Life website and book series (his total lifestyle reboot), blows the lid off conventional life and wellness expectations, and is essential for every person seeking a simpler and better life.

For more information about his publications and services go to: **www.thesimplelifenow.com**.

REFERENCES

21 CFR 101.9 Nutrition labeling of food.

A Calorie Counter. "10 Surprising Foods that Contain Trans Fat." *Acaloriecounter*. Web. 9 APRIL 2011.

"About Fiber." *Wheatfoods*. Web. 5 NOV 2010.

Adams, Mike. "One-Third of American Diet is Junk Food and Soft Drinks: We're Malnourished and Obese at the Same Time." *Naturalnews*. 2 JUNE 2004. Web. 4 NOV 2010.

All About Trans Fats. Washington DC: Weston A. Price Foundation, 2006.

Allbritton, Jen. "Zapping Sugar Cravings." *Wise Traditions* 11.4 (2011): 53-59.

Appleton, Nancy. *Lick the Sugar Habit* (New York: Avery Penguin Putnam,1988).

Astrup, Arne, et al. "Atkins and other low-carbohydrate diets: hoax or an effective tool for weight loss?" *The Lancet* 364.9437 (2004) 897-899.

Atkins, R. C. *Dr. Atkins' New Diet Revolution* (New York: Avon Books, 2002).

Baba, Neal H., et al. "High protein vs high carbohydrate hypoenergetic diet for the treatment of obese hyperinsulinemic subjects." *International Journal of Obesity* 23 (1999):1202-1206.

Baily, Steven. *The Fasting Diet* (McGraw-Hill, 2001).

Bate, Roger and Amir Attaran. "Counterfeit drugs: a growing global threat." *The Lancet* 379 (2012): 685.

Berardi, John Ph.D. "The Importance of Post Workout Nutrition." *Johnberardi.* APR 2002. Web. 23 NOV 2011.

Bercardi, John, and Ryan Andrews. *Nutrition: The Complete Guide* (Carpinteria: International Sports Science Association, 2009).

Bernstein and Willet. "Trends in 24-h urinary sodium excretion in the United States, 1957-2003: a systematic review." *American Journal of Clinical Nutrition* 92.5 (2010): 1172-1180.

Biro, Frank, et al. "Pubertal Assessment Method and Baseline Characteristics in a Mixed Longitudinal Study of Girls." *Pediatrics* 126.3 (2010): 583-590.

Bistrian B.R., et al. "Nitrogen metabolism and insulin requirements in obese diabetic adults on a protein-sparing modified fast." Diabetes 25 (1976): 494–504.

"Biomedicine: The (Political) Science of Salt." The American Association for the Advancement of Science 281.5379 (*Aug 1998*): 898-907.

Booth, Frank W. "Reduced physical activity and risk of chronic disease: the biology behind the consequences." *European Journal of Applied Physiology* 102.4 (2008): 381-390.

Butter is Better. Washington DC: Weston A. Price Foundation, 2010.

Campbell-McBride, Natasha. *Put Your Heart in Your Mouth* (Medinform, 2007).

"Carbohydrates: Good Carbs Guide the Way." *Hsphharvard.* Web. 17 FEB 2011.

Carpenter, Kenneth. *Protein and Energy: A Study of Changing Ideas in Nutrition.* (New York: Cambridge University Press, 1994).

CDC. "2007 National Diabetes Fact Sheet." *Cdc.* 12 MARCH 2010. Web. 10 APRIL 2011.

Centers for Disease Control and Prevention (CDC). "State Indicator on Physical Activity, 2010." CDC. Web. 23 MARCH 2011.

Chek, Paul. *How to Eat Move and Be Healthy* (San Diego, CA: C.H.E.K. Institute, 2009).

Chung, Yoon C., et al. "Protein digestion and absorption in human small intestine." *Gastroenterology* 76.6 (1979): 1415-1421.

References

Collins, Anne. "How we Digest Carbohydrate." *Annecollins*. Web. 5 NOV 2010.

Cordain, Loren, et al. "Origins and evolution of the Western diet: health implications for the 21st century." *American Journal of Clinical Nutrition* 81.2 (2005) 341-354.

Czapp, Katherine. "Against the Grain." *Westonaprice*. 16 JULY 2006. Web. 11 JAN 2011.

Davis, William MD. "Wheat: The Unhealthy Whole Grain." Lef. 1 OCT 2011. Web. 5 JULY 2012.

Di Pasquale, Mauro G. *Amino Acids and Proteins for the Athlete: The Anablolic Edge*. (Boca Raton: CRC Press, 2008).

"Diabetes Statistics." American Diabetes Assoctiation. Web. 31 AUG 2010.

"Diabetes to Double or Triple in U.S. by 2050." *Reuters*. Web. 22 OCT 2010.

"Dietary Supplements: Background Information." *Odsodnih*. National Institute of Health. Web. 9 NOV 2010.

Doheny, Kathleen. "Report: Protein Drinks have Unhealthy Metals." 3 JUNE 2010. Web. 9 NOV 2010.

Dolson, Laura. "What you Need to Know About Complex Carbohydrates." *Lowcarbdiets*. 14 MAR 2009. Web. 2 DEC 2010.

Dyer, Tommy. "Does Fat Make You Fat?" *Themovementdallas*. 16 APR 2009. Web 29 OCT 2010.

Eaton, S. Boyd. "The ancestral human diet: what was it and should it be a paradigm for contemporary nutrition?". *Proceedings of the Nutrition Society* 65.1 (2006): 1-6.

Elliott, Sharon, et al. "Fructose, weight gain, and the insulin resistance syndrome." *American Journal of Clinical Nutrition* 76.5 (2002): 911-922.

Emery, Peter. "Basic metabolism: protein." *Surgery* 27.5 (2009): 185-189.

Engredea News. "CRN consumer survey finds supplement use on the rise." *Newhope360*. 13 March 2012. Web. 19 APRIL 2012.

Enig, Mary G. "Cholesterol and Heart Disease: A Phony Issue." Westonaprice. 30 JUNE 2001. Web. 1 NOV 2010.

Enig, Mary G. *Know Your Fats* (Bethesda: Bethesda Press, 2011).

Enig, Mary G. "Saturated Fat and the Kidneys." *Westonaprice*. 30 SEP 2000. Web. 2 NOV 2010.

Erdmann, Robert. *Fats that can save your life: The critical role of fats and oils in health and disease* (Encinitas, CA: Progressive Health Publishing, 1995).

FDA. "Trans Fat Now Listed with Saturated Fat and Cholesterol on Nutrition Facts Label." *Fda.* 5 April 2011. Web. 9 APRIL 2011.

Furnas, C.C., and S.M. Furnas. *Man Bread and Destiny: The Story of Man and His Food* (New York: New Home Library: 1937).

Graudal, Niels A., et al. "Effects of Sodium Restriction on Blood Pressure, Renin, Aldosterone, Catecholamines, Cholesterols, and Triglyceride: A Meta-analysis." *The Journal of the American Medical Association* 279.17 (1998): 1383-1391.

Grey Neil, and David Kipnis. "Effect of diet composition on the hyperinsulinemia of obesity." *New England Journal of Medicine* 285.15 (1971): 827–831.

Gussow, Joan Dye, and Sharon Akabas. "Are we really fixing up the food supply?" *Journal of the American Dietetic Association* 93.11 (1993): 1300-1304.

Hackney, KJ, et al. "Timing Protein intake increases energy expenditure 24 h after resistance training."

Medicine and Science in Sports and Exercise 42.5 (2010): 998-1003.

Hatfield, Frederick. *Fitness: The Complete Guide* (Carpinteria: International Sports Science Association, 2010).

Hite, Adele H., et al. "In the Face of Contradictory Evidence: Report of the Dietary Guidelines for Americans Committee." *Nutrition Journal* 26.10 (2010): 915-924.

Hobel, Bart. "Sugar on the brain: Study shows sugar dependence in rats." *Princetonedu.* 20 JUNE 2002. Web. 10 FEB 2011.

Hooper L., et al. "Systematic review of long term effects of advice to reduce dietary salt in adults." *British Medical Journal* 325.7365 (2002): 628.

Horne, Benjamin D., et al. "Usefulness of Routine Periodic Fasting to Lower Risk of Coronary Artery Disease in Patients Undergoing Coronary Angiography." *American Journal of Cardiology* 102.7 (2008): 814-819.

"Hunger and Satiety." *Zeroinginonhealth.* Web. 18 NOV 2010.

Jakicic, John M., et al. "Effect of Exercise on 24-Month Weight Loss Maintenance in Overweight Women." *Archive of Internal Medicine* 168.14 (2008): 1550-1559.

Jaminet, Paul Ph.D, Sou-Ching Jaminet, Ph.D. *Perfect Health Diet: Four Steps to Renewed Health, Youthful Vitality, and Long Life* (Cambridge: YinYang Press, 2010).

Jordan, Jo. " USA = Processed Food Nation The harmful Effects of Eating Processed Foods." *Puristat.* Web. 29 OCT 2010.

Kaneshiro, Neil. "Trans Fatty Acids." *Nlmnih.* 2 JULY 2009. Web. 26 OCT 2010.

Katzmarzyk, Peter, et al. "Sitting Time and Mortality from All Causes, Cardiovascular Disease, and Cancer." *Medicine & Science in Sports & Exercise* 41.5 (2009): 998-1005.

Kellock, Brian. "Fiber Man: *The Life Story of Dr. Denis Burkitt* (Lion Publishing Corporation, 1985).

Kovacs, Betty. "Fiber." *Medicinenet.* Web. 5 NOV 2010.

Kummerow, Fred, et al. "Effects of trans fatty acids on calcium influx into human arterial endothelil cells."

American Journal of Clinical Nutrition 70.5 (1999): 832-838.

Kubetin, Sally K. "Demand Swells for Sports Supplements." *Family Practice News* 32.4 (2002): 1.

Larkin, Marilynn. "Little agreement about how to slim down the USA." *The Lancet* 360.9343 (2002): 1400.

Lipinski, Lori. "Replacing Refined Sugars with Natural Sugars One Step at a Time." *Westonaprice.* 10 AUG 2002. Web. 27 SEP 2010.

Litonjua, Augusto A., and Gold, Diane R. "Asthma and obesity: Common early-life influences in the inception of disease." *The Journal of Allergy and Clinical Immunology 121.5 (2008) 1075-1084.*

Keys, Ancel. "Coronary heart disease in seven countries." *Nutrition* 13.3 (1997): 249).

Martin, William F, et al. "Dietary protein intake and renal function." *Nutrition and Metabolism* 2.25 (2005).

Mast, Carlotta. "GAO: Supplements and drugs from China lack regulatory oversight." *Newhope360.* 8 NOV 2010. Web. 19 APRIL 2012.

Masterjohn, Chris. "Essential Fatty Acids." *Wise Traditions* 11.3 (2010): 18-31.

McGuff, Doug and John Little. *Science: A Research Based Program to Get the Results You Want in 12 Minutes a Week* (Northern River Productions, 2009).

McWilliams, James. "China, America and melamine." *Nytimes*. 16 OCT. 2008. Web. 26 JUNE 2012.

Mercola, Joseph D.O. "Add This Seasoning to your Food Daily – Despite What your Doctor Says." 20 SEP 2011. Web. 23 SEP 2011.

Mercola, Joseph D.O. "Lower Your Carb and Lower Your Insulin Levels." *Rheumatic*. Web. 27 SEP 2010.

Mercola, Joseph D.O. "Simple Tip to Radically Increase Your Cellular Energy Production." *Mercola*. 30 SEP 2011. Web. 1 OCT 2011.

Mercola, Joseph D.O. "This One Thing is the Highest Risk for Diabetes." *Mercola*. 16 SEP 2011. Web. 29 SEP 2011.

Mercola, Joseph D.O. "Our Ancestors Didn't Die of Cancer." *Mercola*. 23 SEP 2011. Web. 29 SEP 2011.

Milton, Katharine. "Hunter-gatherer diets—a different perspective." *American Journal of Clinical Nutrition* 71.3 (2000): 665-667.

Mikus Catherine R., et al. "Lowering Physical Activity Impairs Glycemic Control in Healthy Volunteers." *Medicine & Science in Sports & Exercise*, 2011; DOI: 10.1249/MSS.0b013e31822ac0c0.

Monastyrsky, Konstantin. *Fiber Menace* (Ageless Press, 2005).

Moyer, Melinda. "It's Time to End the War on Salt." *Scientific American*. 8 JUL 2011. Web. 23 SEP 2011.

Myths & Truths About Cholesterol. Washington DC: Weston A. Price Foundation, 2010.

Natural Products Insider. "Supplement Sales Surge in Recession." *Naturalproductsinsider*. 13 JAN 2011. Web. 19 APRIL 2012.

Nestle, Marion. *What to Eat* (New York: North Point Press, 2007).

Newton, Paul, et al. "Counterfeit anti-infective drugs." *The Lancet*. 6.9 (2006): 602-613.

Nienhiser, Jill C. "How to Avoid Genetically Modified Foods." *Westonaprice*. Spring 2008. Web. NOV 2010.

Norman, James. "Diabetes: What is Insulin." *Endocrineweb*. 13 OCT 2010. Web. 27 OCT 2010.

Nutrition Business Journal. "NBJ Supplement Business Report." *Newhope360*. 1 SEP 2011. Web. 19 APRIL 2012.

"Nutrient Data Laboratory." *Usdagov*. Web. 10 DEC 2010.

References

O'Keefe, James H., et al. "Achieving Hunter-gatherer Fitness in the 21st Century: Back to the Future." *The American Journal of Medicine* 123.12 (2010): 1082-1086.

Ollberding, Nicholas J, et al. "Food Label Use and Its Relation to Dietary Intake among US Adults." *Journal of the American Dietetic Association*. 110.8 (2010): 1233-1237.

"Omega-3 Fatty Acids: Fact Sheet." *Webmd*. Web. 25 OCT 2010.

"Omega-6 Fatty Acids." *Omega6*. Web. 25 OCT 2010.

Pennington, A.W. "Treatment of Obesity with Calorically Unrestricted Diets." *American Journal of Clinical Nutrition* 1 (1953): 343-348.

Pennington Biomedical Research Center. "Obesity and the Heart." Newsletter #63 (2009).

Peptide Guide. "Amino Acids." *Peptideguide*. Web. 8 MARCH 2011.

Perkins, Cynthia. "The Hidden Dangers of Sugar Addiction." *Holistichelp*. Web. 27 SEP 2010.

Peterson, Dan. "The Sugar Generation and Dental Health." *Dentalgentlecare*. Web. 27 SEP 2010.

Phillips, Bill. *Sports Supplement Review* (Golden: Mile High, 1997).

"Physical Activity and Cancer." *Macmillan*. Web. 14 AUG 2011.

Pollan, Michael. In Defense of Food (England: Penguin, 2008).

Pollan, Michael. *Omnivore's Dilemma* (England: Penguin, 2007).

Powell, Michael. "Assessing the Benefit of Protein Supplementation." *Journal of the American Medical Directors Association* 12.3 (2011): B6.

Pressfield, Steven. *The War of Art* (New York: Warner Books, 2003).

Price, Weston A. *Nutrition and Physical Degeneration* (Price-Pottenger Nutrition Foundation, 2009).

"Proposed Dietary Guidelines for Americans Sharply Debated." *Metabolismsociety*. Web. 6 SEP 2010.

"Psychological Benefits of Exercise." *Appliedsportspsych*. Web. 1 NOV 2010.

Rankin, Janet W. "Role of Protein in Exercise." *Clinics in Sports Medicine* 18.3 (1999): 499-511.

Richetto, David. "Advanced security prevents counterfeit products." *Edn*. 3 NOV 2011. Web. 19 APRIL 2012.

Rodin, J. "Insulin levels, hunger, and food intake: an example of feedback loops in body weight regulation." *Journal of Health Psychology* 4.1 (1985): 1-24.

Rosch, Paul. "The Emperor's New Clothes: Aggressive New Guidelines for Prehypertension." *Westonaprice*. 10 DEC 2003. Web. 24 FEB 2011.

Rosedale, Ron. *The Rosedale Diet* (New York: Harper Collins, 2004).

Salatin, Joel. *Folks This Ain't Normal* (New York: Hachette Book Group, 2011).

Saltos E, Davis C, et al. "Using Food Labels To Follow the Dietary Guidelines for Americans: A Reference - Agriculture Information Bulletin Number 704." *Usda*. 1994. Web. 8 APRIL 2011

Sanuth, Sarah. "The Danger of White Flour." *Helium*. Web. 27 SEP 2010.

Schlosser, Eric, et al. Food Inc. (New York: PublicAffairs, 2009).

Schwarzenegger, Arnold. *The New Encyclopedia of Modern Body Building* (New York: Simon&Schuster, 1998).

Selinger, Susan. "Is Fasting Healthy." Webmd. 1 FEB 2007. Web. 10 APRIL 2011.

Simon GE, Ludman EJ, Linde JA et al. "Association between obesity and depression in middle-aged women." *Gen Hosp Psychiatry*. 30.1 (2008): 32-39.

Simonsick, E., et al. "Just Get Out the Door! Importance of Walking Outside the Home for Maintaining Mobility: Findings from the Women's Health and Aging Study." Journal of the American Geriatrics Society 53 (2005): 198-203.

Singer, Natasha. "Ingredients of Shady Origins, Posing as Supplements." Nytimes. 27 AUG 2011. Web. 9 APRIL 2012.

Stein, Karen. High-Protein, Low-Carbohydrate Diets: Do They Work? *Journal of the American Dietetic Association* 100.7 (2000): 760-761.

Strandberg, Timo E. "A further look at obesity." *The Lancet* 376.9747 (2010): 1144.

"Study Finds Traces of Drugs in Drinking Water in 24 Major U.S. Regions." *Foxnews*. 10 MAR 2008. Web. 7 NOV 2010.

Sturman, Max. *No Sugar No Flour Will Give Me The Power* (San Diego: Do It Naturally Foundation, 2005).

"Super Market Facts: Industry Overview 2006." Food Marketing Institute. Web. 6 SEP 2010.

Taubes, Gary. *Good Calories, Bad Calories* (New York: Random House, 2007).

Taubes, Gary. *Why We Get Fat and What To Do About It.* (Toronto: Random House, 2011).

"The Framingham Heart Study." *Framingham*, Web. 12 FEB 2011.

"Three Screen Report Q1 2010." *Nielsen.* Web. 21 DEC 2010.

Tipton et al. "Timing of amino acid-carbohydrate ingestion alters anabolic response of muscle to resistance exercise." *American Journal of Physiology Endocrinology and Metabolism* 281.2 (2001): 197-206.

"Understanding the Importance of Hydration." Extremenutrition. Web. 10 OCT 2010.

United States Department of Agriculture "Food Guide Pyramid." Usda. Web. 17 FEB 2011.

U.S. Department of Agriculture. "Is Total Fat Consumption Really Decreasing." *Nutritional Insights* (1998): 1-2.

United States Department of Agriculture and United States Department of Health and Human Services. "Report of the Dietary Guidelines Advisory Committee on the Dietary Guidelines for Americans, 2010." *Cnppusda* 15 JUNE 2010. Web. 23 NOV 2010.

United States Food and Drug Administration. "Dietary Supplements." *Fda.* 1 MAY 2012. Web. 28 MAY 2012.

United States Food and Drug Administration. "Generally Recognized as Safe (GRAS)." *Fda.* 10 JUNE 2011. Web. 10 SEPT 2011.

United States Food and Drug Administration. "How to Understand and Use the Nutritional Facts Label." *Fda.* NOV 2004. Web. 7 APRIL 2011.

United States Food and Drug Administration. "Melamine Pet Food Recall of 2007." *Fda.* 29 NOV 2010. Web. 19 APRIL 2012.

United States Food and Drug Administration. "Overview of Dietary Supplements." *Fda.* 16 OCT 2009. Web. 26 JUNE 2012.

Walrand, Stéphane S., et al. "Insulin regulates protein synthesis rate in leukocytes from young and elderly healthy humans." *Clinical Nutrition* 24.6 (2005): 1089-1098.

Wedro, Benjamin. "Lowering Your Cholesterol." *Medicinenet.* Web. 27 OCT 2010.

Wen, Chi Pang, et al. "Minimum amount of physical activity for reduced mortality and extended life expectancy: a prospective cohort study." *The Lancet* 372.9648 (2008): 1473-1483.

William, Connor. "The Importance of Overweight." *Archives of Internal Medicine* 100.1 (1957): 174.

William, Lynne. "What is Olestra." *Wisegeek*. Web. 4 APRIL 2011.

"What is insulin." *Medicalnewstoday*. Web 10 FEB 2011.

Zhao G, Ford ES, Li C et al. "Waist circumference, abdominal obesity, and depression among overweight and obese U.S. adults: National Health and Nutrition Examination Survey 2005-2006." *BMC Psychiatry*. 11.1 (2011): 130.